Praise for *Longevity Nation*

"Michael Clinton stands at the vanguard of a new social movement: longevity. He is both a leader of, and evangelist for, those roaring into the second half of their lives. Through his work, he's discovered the men and women who are foundational to the movement. And in *Longevity Nation*, he introduces us to them, revealing in fascinating detail how these people are reshaping our future lives. Long after you've finished the book, you'll still be thinking about their bold ideas. They will leave you reassured and inspired."

—**Michael Sebastian**, editor in chief of *Esquire*

"Get a wide-angle lens on the implications of our longer lives, and why this should be on the top of everyone's minds. This book will tell you resources you already want to know about and expand one's view to issues you are glad you learned about. This big picture is a valuable overview of the state of transition to a positive longevity society and an immensely enjoyable journey on the full range of issues and opportunities associated with longevity. An important view for individuals, business, education, and government to share toward how we plan and transformational opportunities awaiting."

—**Linda P. Fried, MD, MPH**, director, Butler Columbia Aging Center; professor, epidemiology and medicine; and dean emerita, Mailman School of Public Health Columbia University

"Michael Clinton is at the forefront of the global longevity movement, reimagining what's possible as we live longer lives. He brings together holistic thought leadership across key intersections from beauty and wellness to health and wealth, forming a powerful new narrative for the second half of life, one defined not by age, but by vitality, purpose, and possibility."

—**Justin Boxford**, global brand president, Estée Lauder

"Following up on his bestselling book *Roar*, longevity thought-leader Michael Clinton is back with *Longevity Nation*, a ground-breaking analysis of the strides we have made around living stronger, longer, and the vast, untapped opportunities that remain in the areas of policy, medicine, advertising, and beyond. Leveraging the knowledge and experience of the top scientists, innovators, marketers, and thinkers, this deeply necessary book makes the strongest possible case for reframing the cultural conversation around aging, while offering actionable advice for anyone looking to supercharge the second half of their life."

—**Lucy Kaylin**, editorial director, *Hearst Magazines*

"Michael Clinton masterfully weaves together stories from visionary entrepreneurs, researchers, and communities who are turning demographic challenges into breakthrough opportunities, revealing how forward-thinking leaders are building infrastructure for a world where living to 100 becomes the norm. For anyone seeking to understand and capitalize on the most significant societal shift of our time, *Longevity Nation* is essential reading."

—**Laura L. Carstensen**, PhD, professor of psychology,
Fairleigh S. Dickinson Jr. Professor in Public Policy,
and founding director, Stanford Center on Longevity

"For anyone curious about how longer lives are reshaping who we are and how we live, *Longevity Nation* is the essential guide. Written by Michael Clinton, a gifted storyteller and an aspirational role model for embracing longevity with intention and purpose, the book is both intellectually engrossing and personally transformative."

—**Seth Green**, dean of Graham School, University of Chicago

"*Longevity Nation* recasts aging as a growth strategy, showing how talent, innovation, and agetech translate longer lives into shared prosperity. Clinton offers a clear, optimistic roadmap with real examples we can deploy now to unlock productivity, resilience, and opportunity."

—**Katy Knox**, president, Bank of America Private Bank

"Michael Clinton sees a future of longevity with unprecedented possibilities for health, happiness, innovation, and prosperity. But to realize his vision of longer and better lives, attitudes and expectations about aging must change. Opportunities must be widely shared. Clinton's compelling *Longevity Nation* is a road map and call to action. To realize a brighter future for ourselves and the generations that follow, each of us has a role to play and work to be done."

—**Paul Irving**, senior advisor, Milken Institute; distinguished scholar
in residence, University of Southern California
Leonard Davis School of Gerontology

How to Use:

 INFUSED OIL: Turmeric root (the rhizome) can be gently warmed in a carrier oil to create an infused warming massage oil. Dried rhizome is best for infusion to avoid mold. But be warned—turmeric oil will stain skin and clothing bright yellow.

 TINCTURE: 1 part fresh herb to 2 parts 95% alcohol, or 1 part dried herb to 5 parts 50–60% alcohol. Use to address chronic inflammation and joint and muscle pain, and as a bile stimulant to improve sluggish liver and digestive issues.

 TEA: To make a decoction, gently simmer 2–3 slices fresh turmeric root in 1 cup hot water for 10–15 minutes. To make tea, steep 1 teaspoon dried root per 1 cup hot water for 10 minutes. Used to reduce inflammation, to improve mood and circulation, and to aid in digestion.

 POULTICE AND COMPRESS: Grated turmeric can be applied as a poultice to encourage circulation and reduce localized inflammation. Warm compresses can be made from turmeric tea and applied to sore muscles and joints.

⚠ General Safety:

TOPICAL USE: Well tolerated by most people, but those with sensitive skin may have irritation, redness, or burning with use. Avoid use on broken skin or open wounds. Turmeric stains clothing and skin but lightens when washed.

INTERNAL USE: Generally safe in culinary and tea amounts for most adults and children. May cause mild stomach upset, diarrhea, or nausea in some individuals, especially in high doses. Avoid large doses if you have gallstones, bile duct obstruction, or bleeding disorders, or if you are pregnant or nursing. Considered safe in moderate tea and culinary amounts for pregnant or nursing women, though.

GOOD TO KNOW:

Curcumin is the active compound in turmeric. It is poorly absorbed unless paired with black pepper or fat. Be careful with topical applications, as turmeric will stain clothing and skin bright yellow!

Valerian Root

Valeriana officinalis
Perennial in zones 4–9

Valerian is a tall, fragrant perennial with clusters of white to pale pink flowers, long used as a natural sedative and sleep aid. Its root is the primary medicinal part, valued for calming the nervous system and supporting rest.

Medicinal Properties:

TOPICAL: Not commonly used externally.

INTERNAL: Sedative and nervine; promotes sleep, especially for difficulty falling asleep. Antispasmodic; treats nervous restlessness.

ENERGETIC: Cooling, moistening.

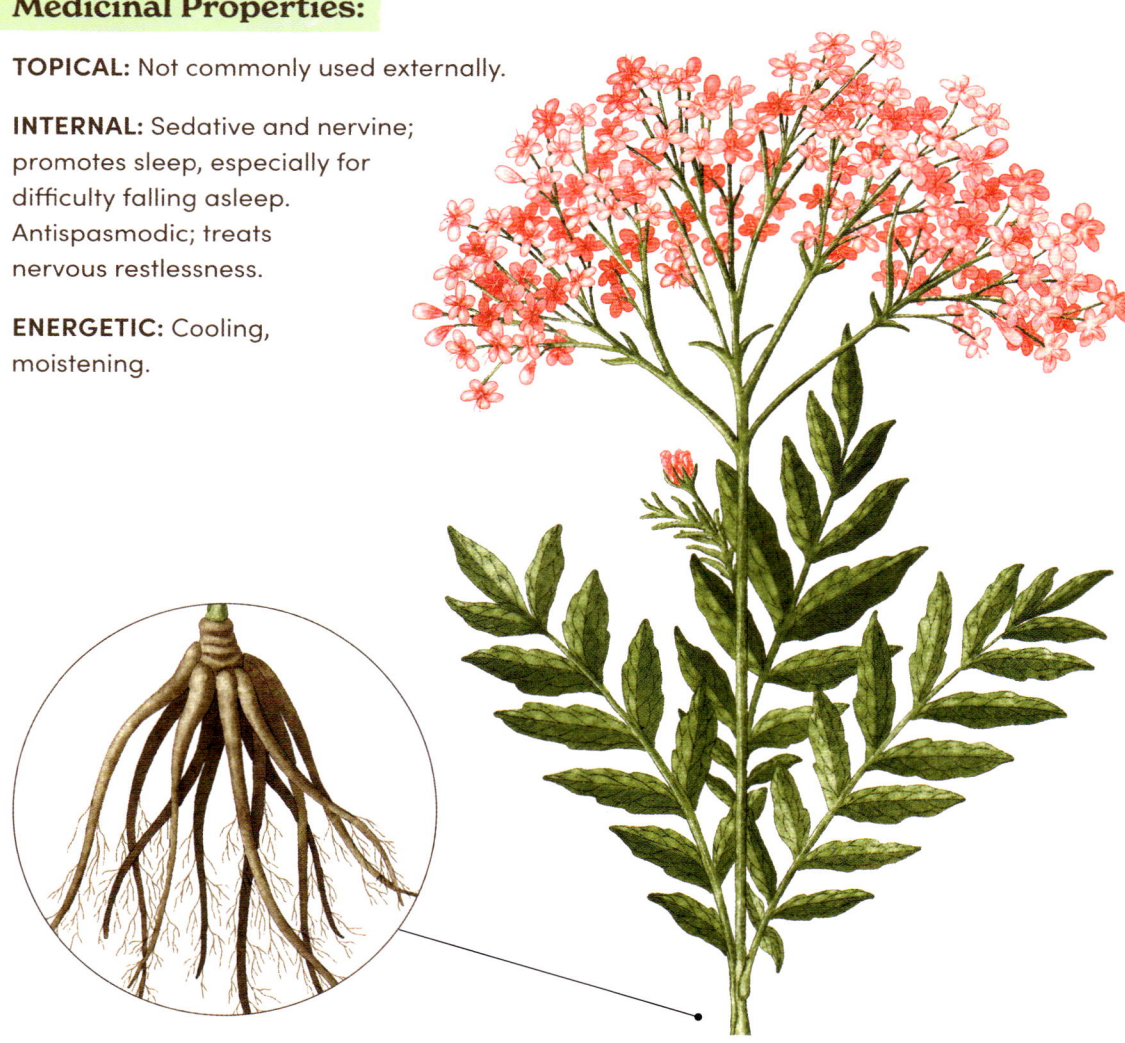

How to Grow:

 WHEN TO PLANT: Sow seeds in spring after last frost, or start indoors 6–8 weeks before transplanting. Can also be propagated by root division in spring or fall.

 GROWS BEST FROM: Seed or root division. Seeds need light to germinate. Sow on the surface of moist soil. Germination can take from 7–21 days under ideal conditions but may take up to 28 days. Once plants have been established for 1–2 seasons, you can dig up the root crown in the dormant months and separate chunks of it to propagate and replant to make more plants.

 SUN AND SOIL NEEDS: Full sun to partial shade. Rich, moist loam and consistent moisture are preferred. Valerian thrives in garden beds near water or damp meadows.

 VARIETIES TO TRY: *Valeriana officinalis*, *Valeriana wallichii*, and *Valeriana sitchensis*.

 SPACING: Space plants 12–18" apart. Clumps spread as roots mature, but overall this plant is relatively low growing and compact when not in bloom. Once flowers bloom, valerian root can shoot up to 4–5' tall.

 BLOOM TIME: Seedlings grow slowly at first and may take 8–10 weeks before they are sturdy enough to transplant outdoors. Plants establish roots and foliage but usually don't produce harvestable roots in the first year.

 HARVESTING TIPS: You can harvest a few leaves for teas or poultices in the first year, but the root should be left intact until the fall of the second year (18–24 months after sowing). This is when medicinal compounds are strongest.

GOOD TO KNOW:

Valerian root has a distinct odor that is sometimes described as "earthy" or like "old socks," which may be off-putting.

How to Use:

 INFUSED OIL: Fresh or dried aerial parts (flowers, stems, and leaves) can be infused for skin-healing salves.

 TINCTURE: 1 part fresh root to 2 parts 65–70% alcohol, or 1 part dried herb to 5 parts 40–50% alcohol. (Keep in mind that dried herb tinctures of valerian can be extra sedating.) Used for calming the nervous system, promoting rest, relieving tension headaches, and easing menstrual cramps.

 TEA: To make a decoction, simmer 1 teaspoon dried root in 1 cup hot water for 10 minutes. Best used as part of a blend, since flavor is strong.

 POULTICE AND COMPRESS: Not typically used as a poultice or compress.

General Safety:

TOPICAL USE: Rarely used externally.

INTERNAL USE: Generally safe for short-term use. May cause grogginess or vivid dreams in some people. A small percentage of people may feel stimulated instead of relaxed. Not recommended for pregnant and nursing women due to lack of safety studies.

HERBALIST TIP:

Because of its off-putting smell, valerian is commonly dried and packed into capsules as a modern herbal supplement. It works best when taken consistently for 1–2 weeks rather than as an occasional sleep aid. If it makes you groggy in the morning, try lowering the dose or combining it with milder nervines, like chamomile or lemon balm.

Violet

Viola odorata
Perennial in zones 4–9 (variety dependent)

Violets are small, shade-loving plants with heart-shaped leaves and delicate purple, white, or yellow flowers. Both the leaves and flowers are medicinal and traditionally used as cooling, moistening remedies for the skin, lungs, and lymphatic system.

Medicinal Properties:

TOPICAL: Violet leaves soothe dry, inflamed, or irritated skin. Poultices or infused oils are used for eczema, rashes, wounds, and breast tenderness.

INTERNAL: Mild nervine relaxant, antispasmodic that can help ease a cough, expectorant, gentle lymphagogue, gentle emmenagogue, demulcent that can help soothe a sore throat, and bitter tonic.

ENERGETIC: Cooling, moistening.

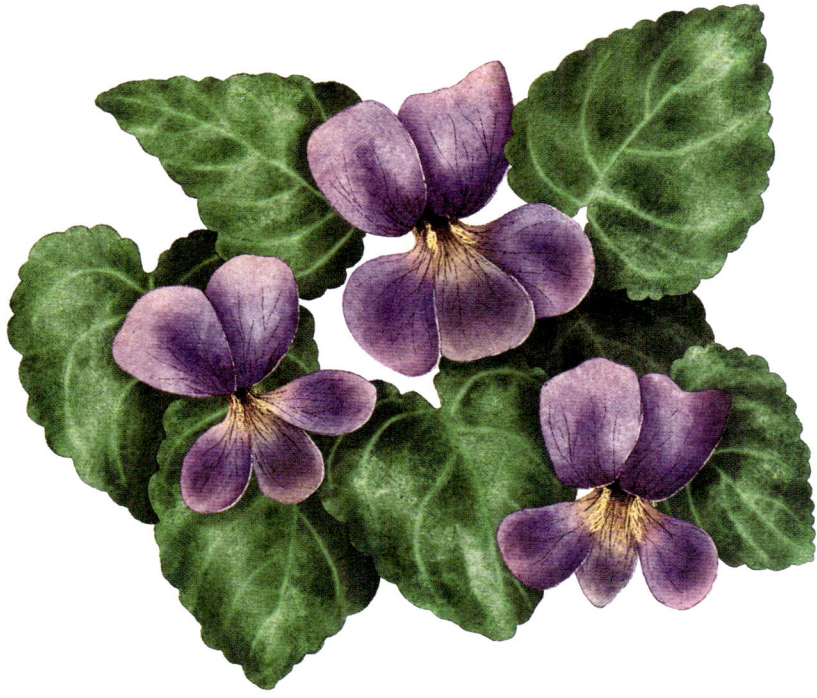

How to Grow:

 WHEN TO PLANT: Sow seeds outdoors in fall (they need natural cold stratification) or indoors in spring after 4–6 weeks of cold stratification in the fridge. Transplant outdoors after frost danger passes, when seedlings have 2–3 sets of true leaves.

 GROWS BEST FROM: Seed or root division. Violets also spread naturally by runners and self-seeding. Violets can be dug up and divided from the root systems to replant elsewhere to make more plants.

 SUN AND SOIL NEEDS: Partial shade to dappled sun. Prefers rich, moist, loamy soil that mimics woodlands edges.

 VARIETIES TO TRY: Sweet violet and heartsease (also called Johnny-jump-up).

 SPACING: Space plants 6–12" apart. Most common violets grow 4–8" tall and form clumps 6–12" wide that can spread over time through rhizomes. Acts as a ground cover in patches under shrubs, fruit trees, or woodland gardens. Container friendly.

 BLOOM TIME: If started early indoors, young plants need 8–12 weeks from germination to reach transplant size. Once planted, violets take time to settle in—in total, it can take plants 4–6 months to grow from seed to having usable leaves and more than a year from seed to producing flowers.

 HARVESTING TIPS: Leaves can be gathered regularly throughout the growing season once established. Flowers are best harvested fresh in early spring when blooms appear (March through May, depending on the climate).

GROWING TIP:

If you want faster access to flowers and leaves, propagating violets from root divisions or runners (rather than seeds) will give you a harvest in the first year instead of waiting two.

How to Use:

 INFUSED OIL: Fresh or dried leaves can be infused in olive or sunflower oil for rashes, eczema, breast massage, or tender skin.

 TINCTURE: 1 part fresh herb to 2 parts 40–50% alcohol, or 1 part dried herb to 5 parts 40% alcohol. Used for lymphatic support and gentle calming. Fresh tincturing captures more of the demulcent moistening qualities of this herb.

 TEA: Steep 1–2 teaspoons dried leaves and flowers, or 1 heaping teaspoon chopped fresh leaves and flowers, per 1 cup hot water for 10–15 minutes. Useful for coughs, sore throats, or mild stress.

 POULTICE AND COMPRESS: Crushed fresh leaves can be applied as a poultice to treat inflamed skin, swollen glands, or minor wounds. A cooled compress made with violet leaves and flowers can provide similar benefits.

 SYRUP: Fresh flowers can be made into a calming, soothing syrup, often used for children's coughs.

⚠ General Safety:

TOPICAL USE: Generally safe and soothing.

INTERNAL USE: Very safe, even for children and elders, when taken in normal food/tea amounts. Gentle and traditionally considered safe for pregnant women, but should be avoided in high doses of tincture without a practitioner's guidance due to mild emmenagogue properties.

HERBALIST TIP:

In folk tradition, violet leaves were carried as charms for protection and love. Unlike stronger nervines, violets are gentle and child-friendly, making them suitable in syrups or teas for kids.

Yarrow

Achillea millefolium

Perennial in zones 3–9

This hardy, feathery-leaved perennial with flat clusters of white, pink, or yellow flowers has been valued since ancient times for its ability to stop bleeding and support overall resilience.

Medicinal Properties:

TOPICAL: Astringent. Helps stop bleeding, closes minor wounds, speeds tissue repair, and soothes inflammation, bruises, and rashes.

INTERNAL: Bitter digestive aid, supporting liver and gallbladder function. Gently stimulates appetite. Diaphoretic that induces sweating to help reduce fevers and cool the body. Helps ease menstrual cramps and regulates cycle.

ENERGETIC: Cooling, drying.

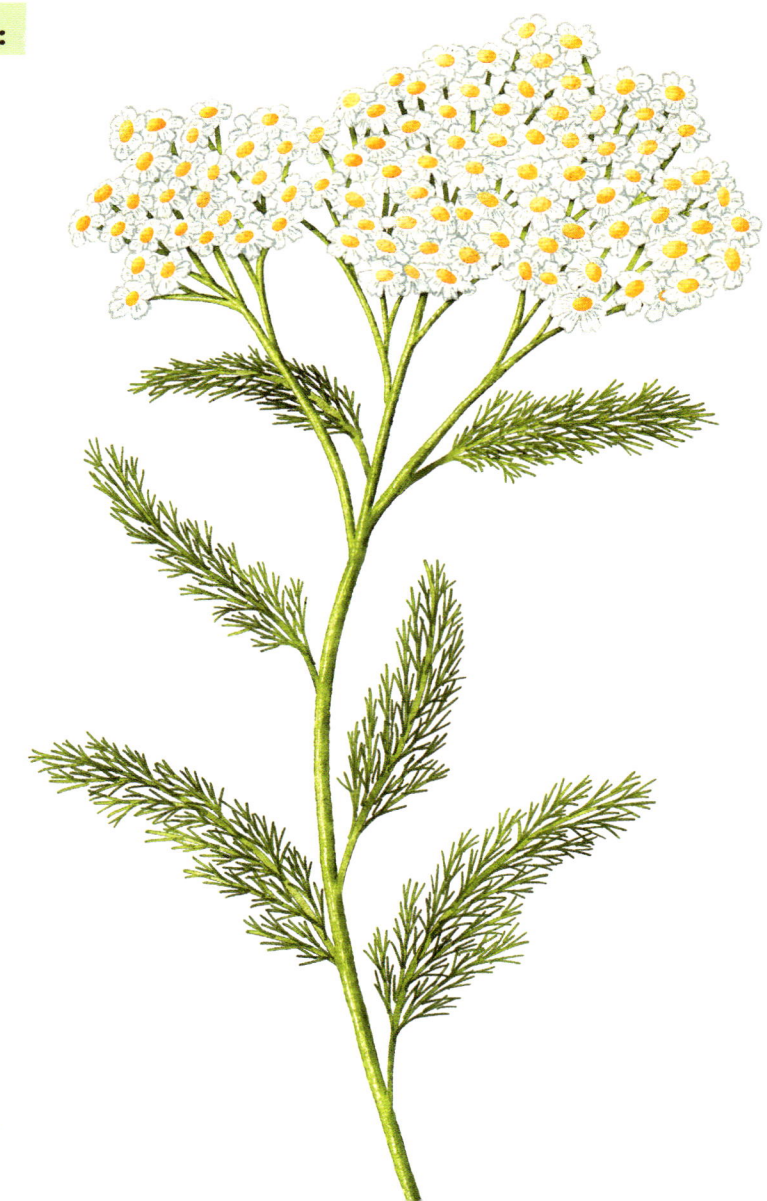

How to Grow:

 WHEN TO PLANT: Start indoors from seed 6–8 weeks before last frost, or direct sow in spring after danger of frost has passed.

 GROWS BEST FROM: Seed, transplant, or root division. Yarrow establishes quickly from division and spreads easily. Yarrow can spread via underground runners, and new shoots will pop up each season that can be dug up and moved into another area to make more plants. Seeds are small, so sprinkling them onto the surface of the soil can aid in germination.

 SUN AND SOIL NEEDS: Full sun, 6–8 hours or more. Tolerates poor, sandy, or dry soils. Very drought tolerant once established.

 VARIETIES TO TRY: Wild yarrow, paprika, Cerise Queen, and yellow yarrow.

 SPACING: Space plants 12–18" apart to allow for vigorous spread. Yarrow will quickly fill in gaps and naturalize via underground rhizomes. Yarrow has been used as a grass alternative in some regions because of its evergreen nature, but keep in mind that it can reach 3' tall when blooming.

 BLOOM TIME: 90–120 days from seed to first flowers.

 HARVESTING TIPS: Leaves can be harvested once the plant is established in its first season, but wait until the second year for strongest yields. Flowers are the best when harvested at full bloom.

GROWING TIP:

Yarrow attracts pollinators and beneficial insects to the garden. Though often seen as a wild plant, cultivated yarrow offers consistent potency and vibrant flowers.

How to Use:

 INFUSED OIL: Freshly wilted or dried leaves can be infused into oils, salves, and balms for topical use.

 TINCTURE: 1 part dried aerial parts to 5 parts 40% alcohol, or 1 part fresh aerial parts to 2 parts 95% alcohol. Used primarily for fever reduction and circulatory support internally.

 TEA: Steep 1–2 teaspoons dried leaves, or 2 tablespoons fresh chopped leaves, per 1 cup hot water, covered, for 5–10 minutes. Helps with fevers, colds, and digestion.

 POULTICE AND COMPRESS: Chewed or bruised fresh leaves can be applied as a poultice to cuts to stop bleeding. You can also make a warm compress with yarrow tea to ease cramps or sore muscles. A cold compress of fresh yarrow leaves can be applied to infected wounds to reduce inflammation and provide antimicrobial support.

 STEAM INHALATION: Add a handful of fresh flowers to a bowl of hot water. Tent your head with a towel and inhale vapors for 5–10 minutes to address sinus congestion or head colds.

⚠ General Safety:

TOPICAL USE: Safe for most people. Some may experience skin sensitivity.

INTERNAL USE: Generally safe in tea or tincture amounts. Yarrow should be avoided in large doses during pregnancy, as it may stimulate uterine contractions.

HERBALIST TIP:

Yarrow is sometimes called "nature's bandage" for its quick action in stopping bleeding when leaves are applied directly to wounds. Yarrow tea works best for fevers when sipped hot, as it helps open pores and encourages sweating to naturally cool the body.

Conclusion

As you've seen throughout these pages, herbal medicine doesn't begin with complicated formulas or expensive ingredients but with soil, sunlight, and patience. The most powerful remedies are often the ones growing quietly right outside your door. From the soft petals of calendula that knit skin back together to the fragrant leaves of holy basil that calm the body and lift the spirit, each plant in this book carries centuries of wisdom written into their roots. Learning to grow and use these herbs brings you back to a rhythm of cultivation and balance between nature and your own needs.

When you grow a medicinal herb garden, you begin to pay attention. You notice how chamomile closes its blossoms before it rains, how lemon balm wilts when soil dries too long, and how motherwort hums with bees in late spring. This kind of attention turns gardening into a relationship. Each time you prune, water, or harvest, you participate in the cycle that nourishes both the plants and yourself. The act of tending becomes medicine long before you brew a cup of tea or fill your first bottle of tincture.

Herbalism is not about replacing modern medicine, but about rebuilding connection and agency in how you care for yourself: A cup of mint tea after a long day, a calendula salve on scraped hands, or a tincture of skullcap when your thoughts won't quiet are all small rituals that invite balance and calm. Over time,

those rituals teach trust in the garden, your senses, and your body's innate capacity to heal.

If there's one lesson these fifty herbs offer, it's that healing is rarely a single event. It's a process of tending to soil, to plants, and to self. You may start by planting for beauty or curiosity, but you'll end up cultivating resilience. Herbs like dandelion remind us that strength can come from persistence even in less-than-ideal conditions. Others, like milky oats, show that gentleness can restore what force never could. Every herb has its own temperament, and learning to match them with your own needs is where true herbal wisdom begins.

As you close this book, I hope you feel inspired to not just grow herbs but to grow with them. Let your garden become a classroom, your kitchen a small apothecary, and your daily life a series of small experiments. Keep notes on what thrives, what fails, and what calls you back each season. Over time, you'll develop your own understanding that is rooted in your region, your soil, and your story. That living knowledge is the heart of herbalism.

So dig your hands into the dirt. Watch, taste, and listen. Let the plants remind you that healing is a slow and steady conversation between the earth and everything it sustains, including *you*. Every leaf you harvest, every seed you sow, carries a simple truth: The garden itself is medicine.

Common Ailments and Their Herbal Remedies

Ailment	Herbs That Can Help
Anxiety, stress and nervous tension	Blue vervain, catnip, chamomile, lemon balm, milky oats, motherwort, passion vine, skullcap, valerian root
Arthritis, joint pain	Feverfew, ginger, lavender, lemongrass, turmeric
Bruises, sprains, swelling	Calendula, comfrey, St.-John's-wort, turmeric, yarrow
Circulatory sluggishness, lymph stagnation	Calendula, echinacea, ginger, mugwort, rose hips, self-heal
Cold, flu, general immune support	Echinacea, elderberry, garlic, ginger, nasturtium, oregano, rose hips, sage, self-heal, thyme
Constipation, poor digestion, sluggish liver	Dandelion root, elecampane, fenugreek, ginger, marshmallow root, mugwort, plantain leaf, rosemary, turmeric
Cough (dry), respiratory irritation	Ginger, licorice root, marshmallow root, mullein, peppermint, turmeric, violet
Cough (wet), chest congestion	Anise hyssop, elecampane, horehound, horsemint, mullein, oregano, thyme
Fever reduction, cooling support	Blue cornflower, elderflower, feverfew, lemongrass, mint, roselle hibiscus, self-heal, yarrow
Gas, bloating, indigestion	Anise hyssop, basil, catnip, cilantro (coriander seed), ginger, holy basil, horsemint, lavender, lemon balm, licorice root, marshmallow root, oregano, peppermint/spearmint

Ailment	Herbs That Can Help
Headaches	Feverfew, lavender, lemon balm, mugwort, peppermint, rosemary
Insomnia, sleep disturbances	California poppy, chamomile, lemon balm, passion vine, skullcap, valerian root
Low mood, mild depression	Bacopa, blue vervain, chamomile, holy basil, passion vine, rose, rosemary, St.-John's-wort, turmeric
Menstrual cramps, PMS support	Blue butterfly pea flower, California poppy, chamomile, motherwort, mugwort
Muscle soreness, cramps	California poppy, lavender, lemongrass, mint, mugwort
Nausea, upset stomach	Chamomile, ginger, horehound, lemon balm, lemongrass, mint (peppermint)
Skin inflammation, insect bites and stings	Calendula, chamomile, echinacea, feverfew, lavender, mint, nasturtium, plantain leaf, violet
Sore throat	Anise hyssop, chamomile, licorice, marshmallow root, mint, plantain leaf, rose, sage, self-heal, violet
Urinary issues, fluid retention	Dandelion root, garlic, licorice root, marshmallow root, mullein, nasturtium, roselle hibiscus, oregano
Wounds (minor), scrapes, rashes/burns	Blue cornflower, calendula, lavender, marshmallow root, plantain leaf, self-heal, violet, yarrow

Standard US/Metric Measurement Conversions

VOLUME CONVERSIONS	
US Volume Measure	**Metric Equivalent**
⅛ teaspoon	0.5 milliliter
¼ teaspoon	1 milliliter
½ teaspoon	2 milliliters
1 teaspoon	5 milliliters
½ tablespoon	7 milliliters
1 tablespoon (3 teaspoons)	15 milliliters
2 tablespoons (1 fluid ounce)	30 milliliters
¼ cup (4 tablespoons)	60 milliliters
⅓ cup	90 milliliters
½ cup (4 fluid ounces)	125 milliliters
⅔ cup	160 milliliters
¾ cup (6 fluid ounces)	180 milliliters
1 cup (16 tablespoons)	250 milliliters
1 pint (2 cups)	500 milliliters
1 quart (4 cups)	1 liter (about)
WEIGHT CONVERSIONS	
US Weight Measure	**Metric Equivalent**
½ ounce	15 grams
1 ounce	30 grams
2 ounces	60 grams
3 ounces	85 grams
¼ pound (4 ounces)	115 grams
½ pound (8 ounces)	225 grams
¾ pound (12 ounces)	340 grams
1 pound (16 ounces)	454 grams

OVEN TEMPERATURE CONVERSIONS

Degrees Fahrenheit	Degrees Celsius
200 degrees F	95 degrees C
250 degrees F	120 degrees C
275 degrees F	135 degrees C
300 degrees F	150 degrees C
325 degrees F	160 degrees C
350 degrees F	180 degrees C
375 degrees F	190 degrees C
400 degrees F	205 degrees C
425 degrees F	220 degrees C
450 degrees F	230 degrees C

BAKING PAN SIZES

American	Metric
8 × 1½ inch round baking pan	20 × 4 cm cake tin
9 × 1½ inch round baking pan	23 × 3.5 cm cake tin
11 × 7 × 1½ inch baking pan	28 × 18 × 4 cm baking tin
13 × 9 × 2 inch baking pan	30 × 20 × 5 cm baking tin
2 quart rectangular baking dish	30 × 20 × 3 cm baking tin
15 × 10 × 2 inch baking pan	30 × 25 × 2 cm baking tin (Swiss roll t n)
9 inch pie plate	22 × 4 or 23 × 4 cm pie plate
7 or 8 inch springform pan	18 or 20 cm springform or loose bottom cake tin
9 × 5 × 3 inch loaf pan	23 × 13 × 7 cm or 2 lb narrow loaf or pâté tin
1½ quart casserole	1.5 liter casserole
2 quart casserole	2 liter casserole

Index

Note: Page numbers in **bold** indicate herb profiles (including medicinal properties; growing and using herbs).

H

Harvesting
  techniques for pruning and, 20–21
  tools for drying and, 28
Headaches, herbs for, 217
Hempseed oil, 37
Herbaceous, tender-stemmed herbs, 13, 15, 20–21, 23
Herb and Feather Seasoning, 48
Herb root types, 14
Hibiscus Cooler, Blueberry Mint, 51
Holy basil, 57, 58, 60, **125–27**. *See also* Basil
Honey Lime Cilantro Mint Vinaigrette, 47
Horehound, 32, 41, 58, **128–30**
Horsemint, **131–33**

I

Immune supportive herbs, 57
Immunity herbs, 58
Indigestion. *See* Digestive (calming) herbs
Infused oils. *See specific herbs*
Infused oils, tools for making, 29
In-ground growing, 23–24
Insect bites/stings, herbs for, 217
Insomnia, herbs for, 217

J

Joint pain, arthritis, 216
Jojoba oil, 37

L

Lavender, 24, 36, 41, 57, 58, 60, **134–36**
Leaf spots, 18–19
Lemon balm, 57, 58, 60, **137–39**
  Nut-Free Nasturtium Lemon Balm Pesto, 45
  Soothing Catnip Chamomile Tea, 52
Lemongrass, 60, **140–42**
Licorice root, 32, 58, **143–45**
Liver, sluggish, 216
Location of garden, 22–24
Lymphagogue, defined, 64
Lymph stagnation, 216

M

Marshmallow root, 55, 58, **146–47**, 148
Medicinal herbs, growing, 13–14. *See also specific herbs*
  about: getting started overview, 8–9; overview and summary, 10, 215; this book and, 7
  calculating growing season length, 11–12
  designing gardens, 22–25
  diseases and treatments, 18–19
  goals for, 22
  perennial/biennial/annual defined, 12
  pest control, 16–18
  propagating herbs, 21
  pruning and harvesting techniques, 20–21
  soil requirements, 14–16
  types of herbs, identifying, 13–14
Medicinal properties. *See specific herbs*
Menstrual cramps, herbs for, 217
Milky oats, 57, **148–49**
Mint, 36, 41, 57, 60, **152–54**. *See also* Horsemint
  Blueberry Mint Hibiscus Cooler, 51
  Breathe Deep Cold and Flu Support Tea, 53–54
  Honey Lime Cilantro Mint Vinaigrette, 47
Moistening herbs, 27
Mood (low, mild depression), herbs for, 217
Motherwort, 32, **155–57**
Mucilage, 28
Mugwort, 32, **158–60**
Mullein, 58, **161–63**
Muscle soreness, cramps, 217

N

Nasturtium, **164–66**
Nasturtium, in Nut-Free Nasturtium Lemon Balm Pesto, 45
Nausea, herbs for, 217
Nervine, defined, 64
Nervine/adaptogenic herbs, 57
Nervous tension, stress, anxiety, 216
Nut-Free Nasturtium Lemon Balm Pesto, 45

LONGEVITY NATION

The **People**, **Ideas**, and **Trends** Changing the Second Half of Our Lives

MICHAEL CLINTON

ATRIA BOOKS
New York Amsterdam/Antwerp London
Toronto Sydney/Melbourne New Delhi

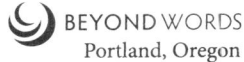
BEYOND WORDS
Portland, Oregon

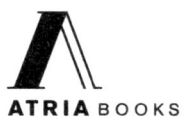

ATRIA BOOKS
An Imprint of Simon & Schuster, LLC
1230 Avenue of the Americas
New York, NY 10020

BEYOND WORDS
1750 S.W. Skyline Blvd., Suite 20
Portland, Oregon 97221-2543
503-531-8700 / 503-531-8773 fax
www.beyondword.com

This publication contains the opinions and ideas of its author. It is intended to provide helpful and informative material on the subjects addressed in the publication. It is sold with the understanding that the author and publisher are not engaged in rendering medical, health, or any other kind of personal professional services in the book. The reader should consult his or her medical, health, or other competent professional before adopting any of the suggestions in this book or drawing inferences from it. The author and publisher specifically disclaim all responsibility for any liability, loss or risk, personal or otherwise, which is incurred as a consequence, directly or indirectly, of the use and application of any of the contents of this book.

Managing Editor: Lindsay S. Easterbrooks-Brown
Editors: Sarah Heilman, Michele Astiani Cohn
Copyeditor: Ashley Van Winkle
Proofreader: Indigo: Editing, Design, and More
Design: Devon Smith
Cover Art: Vecteezy.com
Composition: William H. Brunson Typography Services

First Beyond Words/Atria hardcover edition May 2026

For information about special discounts for bulk purchases, please contact Simon & Schuster Special Sales at 1-866-506-1949 or business@simonandschuster.com.

The Simon & Schuster Speakers Bureau can bring authors to your live event. For more information or to book an event, contact Simon & Schuster Speakers Bureau at 1-866-248-3049 or visit our website at www.simonspeakers.com.

Manufactured in the United States of America

10 9 8 7 6 5 4 3 2 1

Library of Congress Control Number: 2026931389

ISBN: 978-1-58270-962-8
ISBN: 978-1-6680-9729-8 (ebook)

The corporate mission of Beyond Words Publishing, Inc.: *Inspire to Integrity*

Dedicated to those who strive to live a happy, healthy, purpose-driven 100-year life.

Contents

Foreword

Throughout most of human history, average life expectancy was about 20 years. When seventeenth-century British philosopher Thomas Hobbes described life as "nasty, brutish, and short,"[1] life expectancy had reached a mere 38 years. One hundred years later, it had crept up to 42. Progress was glacial, measured in single digits across entire centuries.

Then something extraordinary happened.

By the dawn of the twentieth century, life expectancy in the United States had reached 47 years. By century's end, it had soared to 77—a near-doubling in just one hundred years. We didn't evolve into a hardier species; natural selection had nothing to do with this dramatic transformation. Instead, our twentieth-century ancestors embarked on an unprecedented mission: They built a world to protect young life.

The effort wasn't confined to medical science, although the development of vaccines and antibiotics, along with public health efforts to inoculate the entire population, played critical roles in reducing infant and child mortality. Rather, the increase in longevity reflected a much broader societal effort. Agricultural technologies ensured a steady food supply throughout the year. The public disposal of waste (a.k.a. garbage collection) reduced the spread of contagious diseases. Electricity and electrical power lines allowed for household refrigeration, significantly improving the safety of the food supply. Public education was put in place in every state to teach all children how to read and write.

The private sector played a crucial role in the distribution of life-saving products such as heating and air conditioning, antiseptics, and soap, which became widely accessible. General stores evolved into supermarkets. Pasteurized milk became readily available. Mail-order companies like Sears, Roebuck & Co., and Montgomery Ward distributed heating and cooling products to consumers nationwide. Telephony connected communities, strengthening social ties and letting people get help when needed.

These collective efforts fundamentally transformed how people lived.

Yet as a new demographic reality emerged, alarm bells began to ring. Many people forecast a nightmare scenario: An aging population would create unprecedented burdens for families and institutions. Worker productivity would decline with older employees. Resources would be diverted to elder care, shortchanging children and young families.

But this handwringing misses a fundamental truth. Rather than an impending crisis, longer lives represent an unprecedented chance to re-envision the life course and draw a New Map of Life. More years mean more time to spend with our loved ones and to chase our dreams. Addressing problems and building a longevity nation will not happen by luck or chance. Longevity is at the same time among the greatest opportunities and the greatest challenges of the twenty-first century.

The good news is that some of our most innovative minds— scientists, entrepreneurs, and thought leaders—are pioneering what can be called the "new longevity movement." Like previous social movements addressing women's rights, racial justice, and environmental protection, this movement recognizes the potential that an extended lifespan represents.

In laboratories around the nation, scientists are beginning to identify mechanisms that drive aging and asking whether they can be slowed or even reversed. We stand at the threshold of unlocking the mysteries of aging, identifying factors that allow some individuals to thrive while others succumb to illness and decline. The science is accelerating. There is little doubt that much of what we believe today about aging will be revised or rejected—as is the nature of scientific progress. The exciting reality is that serious inquiry has begun. As my biophysicist father used to say, "The tentative nature of knowledge doesn't speak against science; it is science."

Just as gains in longevity in the twentieth century required more than medical breakthroughs, optimizing longevity in the twenty-first century demands contributions from across society. This book introduces you to experts who span business, education, healthcare, entertainment, and basic research—from entrepreneurs who create products that help people build wealth over extended lifespans, to city planners who design communities for century-long lives, to venture capitalists who fund promising start-ups, to educators who see the need to move from schooled societies to learning societies.

The movement has momentum. Future historians will mark this as a pivotal era in human development. In *Longevity Nation*, Michael Clinton invites you to meet the pioneers leading the charge to create a world that doesn't just accommodate longer lives—but celebrates and maximizes the potential of century-long lifespans.

—Laura L. Carstensen, PhD
Professor of Psychology
Fairleigh S. Dickinson Jr. Professor in Public Policy
Director, Stanford Center on Longevity

Preface

You've probably noticed that the word longevity has become a big part of the global conversation. With advances in medicine and technology, and increased focus on healthier lifestyles, we are in a seismic shift that will lead to longer life expectancies that only a generation ago would have seemed improbable. Throughout the world, doctors, technologists, investors, and leaders in academia, business, entertainment, nonprofits, and more are engaged as the architects of this exciting new longevity era. Their efforts have begun to converge to create a longevity ecosystem of services, products, and ideas to build the new construct for the second half of life. Whether they are designing precision medicine, a new class of longevity drugs, AI robots, new tech-enabled skincare procedures, or more age-friendly cities, they are the longevity innovators of our time. They are creating new workplace models, government policies, and social structures, all to support a world where living to 100 is normalized.

all to support a world where living to 100 is normalized

Some people wonder if it is a good thing to live to that age, but if you ask most people if they want to reach 100, assuming they would still have their mobility and cognitive abilities intact, the answer is a resounding yes.

We're well on the way to that being a reality for many people. Studies around the world suggest that today's 5-year-old will have a 50 percent chance of reaching 100.[1] There are currently 722,000 centenarians in the world, and that number is projected to grow to 25 million or more by the year 2100, according to United Nations data.[2] That growth will have an enormous impact on countries, healthcare systems, social support structures, businesses, and individuals. The work to make the necessary changes is already underway.

From less than a million centenarians to 25 million in just seventy-five years seems like a big jump. But it's not unprecedented. In 1900, the average life expectancy in the United States was 47.[3] The idea of everyone living to 80 seemed preposterous at the time, yet that is the average life expectancy today. So why does 100 seem so far-fetched?

The question is, are we *ready* for the 100-year life?

Many people are. In 2024, the last baby boomers turned 60. For many, even as they reached this milestone, there was a very real awareness that living another thirty or forty years was a real possibility. As the activist generation that challenged many institutions throughout their lives, they have now taken on longevity—living longer, healthier lives—as their new cause. In my book *ROAR: into the second half of your life (before it's too late)*, I identified this group as the Re-Imagineers, the front-runners who are the age innovators among us. Many Generation X individuals are already a part of the movement, and when the first millennials turn 50 in the year 2031, they will join in, swelling the ranks of Americans aged 50 and up to 130 million.[4] These Re-Imagineers are working longer, launching new careers at 60, starting businesses, going back to school, and establishing new relationships. They exclaim that 60 is not the new 40, but rather 60 is the new 60, and 70 is the new 70, and this is what it can look like.

To really get the conversation going, I always suggest that people read Ray Kurzweil, particularly his newest book, *The Singularity Is Nearer*, which discusses what might happen when we merge with AI.[5] It's a fascinating journey into what the future might look like with the combination of AI and the nanotechnology revolution that might allow us to redesign and rebuild, molecule by molecule, our bodies and brains and the world in which we interact. Will we be able, as he suggests, to greatly transcend the current human limit of 122 years with nanorobots patrolling our bloodstreams to detect health issues? Will there be lab-grown organs, 3D bioprinting for organ replacement, and AI brain-augmenting techniques that will allow us to go far beyond our current human capabilities? It's all worth contemplating. If anyone says that such things are not possible, all we have to do is look at the marvels of technology and where it has already taken us in all aspects of our lives. My opinion is that no one really has the answers. We won't know until we know.

There is still a lot of work to do to manifest the changes that we will need to realize the longevity nation of the future. We especially need to ensure that what is created is available to everyone. The professional Re-Imagineers who are building the pathways to make it happen are deep into their work. My goal in this book is to celebrate many of them for their ideas and vision. One hundred years from now, those who come after us may find it curious that we were even talking about the possibility of a 100-year life. They may have already moved on, contemplating how they will be preparing for the 150-year-old life!

Welcome to longevity nation.

Introduction

In 2023, a team and I launched ROAR forward, a joint venture with the Hearst Corporation (where I spent more than twenty years in the magazine company) to focus on the new longevity. Our goal has been to bring data, insights, and content to leaders across all industries about the global longevity movement. So far, we've worked with the highest levels of management at more than fifty companies.

Shortly after forming, ROAR forward commissioned its first major study to get a deeper understanding of this newly emerging cohort. Collaborating with the National Research Group, we conducted a mix of in-depth interviews and surveys of 1,500 people who were 50–70 years old, balanced by age, gender, and ethnicity.[1] We included filters for income and education and certain attitudinal behaviors, allowing us to compare our group to the general population. The objective was to establish the first psychographic profile of this demographic. Our observation was that the boomers who were the original activists on many fronts were now taking on their new cause as the Re-Imagineers—the age innovators who are engaged in rewriting the script for what the second half of life can look like. These people are proactive, curious, engaged, and positive about their post-50 life.

proactive, curious, engaged, and positive

The findings were a breakthrough in that they showed a lot of people in this age group were innovators. One in three identified with the characteristics that identified them as a Re-Imagineer. This validated our belief in the rise of age innovators.

Our research provided some key insights into the changing attitudes, behaviors, and motivations of this group. Eighty-five percent reported that post-50 is the new prime of life. Ninety-five percent said they are coming into that prime energized, motivated, and focused on their next chapters. They reject the default cultural representations of older Americans as having physical and cognitive limitations. They're frustrated about imagery and messaging in media and advertising on this front. Ninety-one percent said they want to see more modern images of what it means to be in their age group. Sixty-two percent said they notice and respond negatively to outdated and stereotypical people their age in advertising, and one in five stopped buying a specific brand product or service because it did not represent or connect to people over 50.

The Re-Imagineers also see retirement as an antiquated idea, an old-fashioned construct that was created when life expectancy was in the early 60s. Sixty-eight percent said that the previous generation's approach to retirement and the second half of life was out of date. This group expects to work longer and in different ways. They see work as a form of enrichment and accomplishment, as well as a way to earn more income. They see the possibility of "post-career" work as a new horizon in their lives. It's true that many may have to work in order to fund a much longer life, but a 2024 Retirement Confidence Survey by the Employee Benefit Research Institute and Greenwald Research found that the majority of retirees who are still working for pay do so because they want to stay active and involved (85 percent) and/or because they enjoy it (80 percent).[2] Furthermore, in our study, sixty-seven percent of individuals reported that they had already started something new.[3]

Working for pay isn't the only way people are finding meaning, though. Whether it is involvement in philanthropy or volunteerism, in the ROAR study, 88 percent reported that it is important to help others and be of service to the community. At this stage of their lives, they have wisdom, experience, knowledge, and a desire to put it to use. Re-Imagineers are viewed as highly influential among their peers, as they inspire others to join the movement of possibilities in the second half of life. While 33 percent of the population of 50-to-70-year-olds might be defined as members of the Re-Imagineer cohort, their appeal is wide, and 74 percent of the general population control group said that they aspired to be like the Re-Imagineers. Obviously, we are in the middle of a particularly powerful social movement.

> **they have wisdom, experience, knowledge, and a desire to put it to use**

Many such social movements have front-runners who are ahead of their time, becoming catalysts for change. For example, the early suffragette movement had Elizabeth Cady Stanton and Susan B. Anthony, and second-wave feminism had Betty Friedan, Shirley Chisholm, and Gloria Steinem. The civil rights movement had W. E. B. Du Bois and Booker T. Washington and later Rosa Parks, Dr. Martin Luther King Jr., Whitney Young, and Roy Wilkins. The early gay rights movement had the Mattachine Society and later Harvey Milk, Henry Gerber, and Bruce Voeller. These social movements created change that forever altered our society and culture.

Today, the world is in the midst of what many call the "new longevity movement," and this time, every human being is affected regardless of gender, race, identity, religion, or politics. This movement got its start decades ago and has continued to grow through the hard work of key new longevity leaders, including the following:

- New longevity pioneers Ken Dychtwald and his wife Maddy founded Age Wave in 1986 to raise awareness of this seismic change.
- Dr. Joseph Coughlin founded the MIT AgeLab in 1999 to improve the quality of life of older people and those who care for them.
- Peter Peterson, former Secretary of Commerce, wrote the seminal book *Gray Dawn: How the Coming Age Wave Will Transform America—and the World* in 2000.

- Dr. Laura Carstensen cofounded the Stanford Center on Longevity in 2007 to focus on the impact that living longer was going to have on the world.
- Dr. David Sinclair, professor of genetics at Harvard and coauthor of *Lifespan: Why We Age—and Why We Don't Have To*, has suggested that the first person who will live to be 150 years old may have already been born.
- Dr. Aubrey de Grey, a British biomedical gerontologist, has made the claim that rejuvenation biotechnology may enable human beings alive today to live longer and even avoid death from age-related causes. While some of his peers question that possibility, who really knows what the future holds?

No matter where you look, you will find Re-Imagineer leadership moving us all forward into the longevity era. They are being joined by everyday Re-Imagineers, individuals who have broken the mold of having to "wind down" or give up on dreams in the second half of their lives. Instead, they are embracing the possibilities that await them as they anticipate living into their 80s, 90s, or longer. These are the people you will learn about and from in the subsequent chapters.

they are embracing the possibilities that await them as they anticipate living into their 80s, 90s, or longer

For example, in chapter 1, you will learn about the work of Laura Carstensen, Jack Rowe, Linda Fried, and others. These Re-Imagineers are committed to finding longevity solutions that will make it possible for everyone to enjoy a healthy and happy extended life.

In chapter 2, we'll discuss the importance of life layering and learn about three Re-Imagineer programs that provide Re-Imagineers with the tools they need to map out the next stages of their lives. In the process, we'll meet a variety of Re-Imagineers, including Chip Conley, Mark Buchanan, and Pamela Corante.

In chapter 3, we'll explore some of the many educational opportunities offered by universities and other academic institutions and discuss how they can help you relaunch your life. As we learn about these programs, we'll also meet some Re-Imagineers who have seized these academic opportunities and completely changed their lives as a result.

Chapter 4 takes a close look at some of the ways workplaces are evolving to retain and support their over-50 talent through age-inclusive cultures, reskilling, and upskilling. This chapter also takes a look at efforts being made by companies and Re-Imagineers around the world to prevent talent drain.

In chapter 5, we'll explore how to launch a new career or become an entrepreneur after age 50. As we do this, we'll meet a number of Re-Imagineers, including Norman Miller, Ron Minutella, and Yolanda Taylor, who pursued their later-in-life career dreams, a process that often involved shifting into an industry that was completely new to them.

Chapter 6 explores the challenges of funding a 100-year life and the importance of financial literacy and planning. It also introduces some key Re-Imagineers who are actively working in this space, discusses the government's role in financial longevity, and describes some international efforts to support people as they age.

Chapter 7 is all about the importance of remaining creative as we age. We'll explore some of the benefits of creativity and learn about a few of the organizations that are providing training and support to older adults who are looking to start or expand their creative journeys. We'll also meet a few Re-Imagineers who have pursued creative endeavors, including Alex Rotas, Alissa Randall, John Kneapler, and Tina Woods.

In chapter 8, we'll discuss how advertising and media have traditionally viewed older adults and how this is beginning to change. We'll also meet some of the people involved in making media a more age-inclusive space, including David Sable, Paul Woolmington, and Stephanie Fierman.

In chapter 9, we'll discuss traveling during the second half of life. The number of travel options specifically targeting older adults is growing to cater to all tastes and budgets, and we'll explore a few of them in detail.

Chapter 10 introduces the exciting world of longevity medicine and describes recent advances in this area. We'll also meet some key Re-Imagineers in this space, including Mark Lachs, Nir Barzilai, and Jennifer Garrison, who are conducting research and making discoveries that are going to help all of us live longer, healthier lives. We'll also take a special look at longevity clinics in Singapore, a country that is leaps and bounds ahead of most others in the longevity space.

Chapter 11 continues the discussion of longevity medicine, with a special focus on how technology, including AI, is changing the game. In this chapter, we'll discuss new research in this intersection of industries, discover some of the recent advances that have been made possible by AI, and meet some of the people driving these advances, including Dr. David Luu, Dr. Wendy Chapman, and Dr. Jennifer Schrack.

Chapter 12 further builds on the discussion of the role technology is playing in longevity health, but shifts the focus to the importance of sleep. We'll begin by discussing the history of sleep science and then explore the relationship between sleep and health in later life. We'll cover some of the technology that is helping people sleep, and then round out the chapter with some simple sleep hacks that anyone can follow.

In Chapter 13, we'll describe the role that diet and exercise play in longevity, and learn from experts in these areas, including Dr. Michael Frederickson and Dr. Gabrielle Lyon. We will finish the chapter with a discussion of the rise of GLP-1 drugs and how they are changing the game.

Chapter 14 explores the link between healthy skin and longevity and introduces new advances in this space. In the process, we'll meet some key Re-Imagineers and researchers in the skincare industry, including Dr. Anne Chang, Dr. Zakia Rahman, Dr. Haideh Hirmand, and Dr. Steve Dayan. We'll also learn about efforts being made by companies like Estée Lauder and L'Oréal to create skincare products that are available to everyone, not just those who can afford the most cutting-edge and experimental technology.

Chapter 15 discusses the importance of maintaining and building new relationships as we age. It introduces key organizations and Re-Imagineers who are working to build community and provide social support to those who need it, and it describes the role that technology and online communities are playing in this process.

In Chapter 16, we continue the discussion of community, but shift the focus to how physical locations are being adapted and updated to get the world "longevity ready." We'll learn about efforts in Singapore, the United Arab Emirates, Japan, the United Kingdom, and elsewhere to promote longevity and accommodate the physical and emotional needs of older adults. The chapter finishes with a discussion of the situation in the United States, which lags behind efforts in many other developed nations.

As you'll learn throughout this book, the combination of everyday people who are part of the Re-Imagineer movement, in tandem with leaders in business, government, and academia, will propel cultures and societies into longevity nations. We are already on our way on a global level. Over the next decade, we will see enormous progress made on multiple fronts that will change how we live and what we think about the second half of life. Like other social movements, this one is being driven by front-runners, the Re-Imagineers, those who see the opportunities in the new longevity movement and are acting on them.

the combination of everyday people who are part of the Re-Imagineer movement, in tandem with leaders in business, government, and academia, will propel cultures and societies into longevity nations

They are the builders of the longevity nation. Older populations are here and fundamentally changing the world. It's not a moment in time; it is a long-term trend that is here to stay.

In the movie *The Graduate*, Mr. McGuire takes young Ben Braddock aside to give him a word of advice for his future: "I just want to say one word to you. . . . Plastics."[4] Channeling that same energy, my advice to people who are looking for a change or new direction is "I just want to say one word to you: *longevity*." The opportunities are endless.

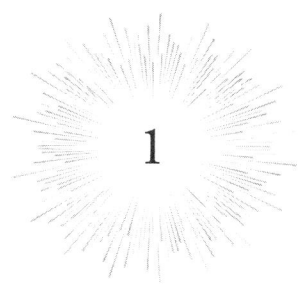

The OG Re-Imagineers of Longevity

While the longevity phenomenon has only recently become part of the global zeitgeist, there has been a longstanding group of thought leaders. Many of them work in academia, the nonprofit sector, government, medicine, and business, and they have been working on innovative solutions and ideas to address the demographic upheaval that is sweeping the globe. They are the OG Re-Imagineers. They have long been committed to the goal of finding longevity solutions that are available to all people, regardless of their socioeconomic status or country of origin. Democratizing healthcare, finding better ways to build financial security, fostering community, and forging intergenerational relationships are consistent themes in their work.

If you'd like a deep dive into an expanded list of the players in the longevity space, you can check out groups like the World Health Organization's "Healthy Ageing 50" leaders who are transforming the world to be a better place to grow older. Other notable lists include the Aging Analytics Agency's "Top-50 Women Longevity Leaders" and "Top-100 Longevity Leaders." The number of longevity leaders across every sector of business, academia, medicine, technology, and more is growing exponentially as the longevity nation expands. Dr. Andrew Huberman, a Stanford neuroscientist and host of the podcast Huberman Lab, is one example of a major voice in the space. Those thought leaders who stimulate new thinking that leads to new discoveries, ideas, and trends will top the lists in future years. Although I cannot cover every longevity leader in this book, here are a few of the OG Re-Imagineers.

Laura Carstensen

Laura Carstensen, PhD, professor of psychology and the Fairleigh S. Dickinson Jr. Professor in Public Policy at Stanford University, is the founding director of the Stanford Center on Longevity (SCL). Carstensen is one of the OGs of the movement (she also graciously agreed to write the foreword to this book). The SCL was founded in 2007, with her colleague Thomas Rando, MD, PhD, a stem cell biologist and professor of neurology. The premise of the center is that life expectancy has increased so rapidly that the world is unprepared. We need to expand medical science to include diseases of old age, rethink social norms that guide us through life, retrofit buildings and homes to accommodate an age-diverse population, and develop technologies that compensate for vulnerabilities that eventually affect us all. As a member of the SCL Advisory Board since 2022, I've witnessed firsthand the incredible work that the Center does. Working with more than 150 Stanford faculty and others, they have had a nearly twenty-year commitment to building on longevity expertise.

"Importantly, we are a center on longevity, not old age," explained Carstensen, adding that "the worlds of work, medicine, education, and lifestyle are all interconnected to enhance how longevity becomes a lifelong effort."[1]

SCL's landmark initiative, the New Map of Life, was developed to reimagine social institutions, norms, and policies that were created when life expectancies were half of what they are today. SCL works closely with industries and businesses. "It is an all-hands, all-sector undertaking requiring the best ideas from the private sector, government, medicine, academia, and philanthropy," said Carstensen.[2]

To get the world ready for a new reality, the map explores the alignment of health spans to lifespans for all populations, especially those affected by poverty, discrimination, and environmental damage. "Age diversity is a net positive for society, as we all go on this journey together," said Carstensen.[3]

With almost twenty years of research, insights, and recommendations, SCL now finds itself in the red-hot center of the longevity movement. In future years, expect them to continue to lead on the subject.

Other major studies on longevity, comparable to Stanford's New Map of Life, include The Global Roadmap for Healthy Longevity, commissioned by the National Academy of Medicine (2022); The World Health Organization's World Report on Ageing and Health (2015); and the subsequent Global Strategy and Action Plan on Ageing and Health (2016–2020). The UN Decade of Healthy Aging (2021–2030), which is being implemented by the World Health Organization (WHO) in collaboration with other UN organizations, is a massive initiative to focus on longer and healthier lives for the growing global population of older people.

The Okinawa Centenarian Study (OCS) began in 1975 and is the longest-running of these longevity studies. It examines more than one thousand centenarians and other selected older people from Okinawa, a Japanese prefecture of 150 islands whose citizens have exceptional longevity.[4] Carried out by the Okinawa Research Center for Longevity Sciences, it looks at a broad range of topics such as activities of daily living, lifestyle habits, medical history, and other health measurements. It continues to bring great insights in the factors that contribute to healthy and longer lives.

The McKinsey Global Institute reported on the implications of the longevity factor and its effect on the world in their 2025 paper *Dependency and Depopulation? Confronting the Consequences of a New Demographic Reality*. Other efforts from the World Economic Forum, the Milken Institute, CoGenerate, the Robert N.

Butler Columbia Aging Center, and more will be covered in later chapters of this book.

———————

Jack Rowe

Dr. Jack Rowe has been in the aging and longevity space for more than 50 years. He has published more than two hundred 200 scientific publications, mostly on the aging process, coauthored the book *Successful Aging* with Robert Kahn, and is recognized as one of the leading voices in the space. He has served as a professor at both Harvard and Stanford Medical Schools and is currently the Julius B. Richmond Professor at Columbia University's Mailman School of Public Health. One of his many past leadership experiences was being president and chief executive officer of Mount Sinai New York Health. "For many years, I felt like Sisyphus pushing the rock up the hill every day only to start from the bottom the next day. It was exceptionally difficult to get traction on research about aging or to attract elite scientists to focus on it," he said, adding that "it was all in the perception of what aging meant then versus today."[5]

> It was exceptionally difficult to get traction on research about aging or to attract elite scientists to focus on it

With his long perspective on the field, Rowe said that there has been a rapid shift in the past several years that is propelling the field forward in exciting ways and changing the focus from disability, disease, and frailty to successful aging. He noted that the emergence of "geroscience" has created exciting developments in biology that are modifying the rate of aging. For example, senescent cells, which are cells that are advanced in age and secrete chemicals that are toxic, are now being treated by senolytic drugs such as metformin and rapamycin. Metformin has been shown to help reduce the harmful effects of senescent cells, and rapamycin is an mTOR inhibitor that can delay the development of cellular senescence.

According to Rowe, the field is now attracting elite scientists who want to study aging with a different perspective. What was once only identified as geriatrics is now expanding into longevity medicine. This new generation of scientists and doctors are attracted to this idea, conducting clinical trials that find new drugs and meaningful solutions for longevity. Examples include biomarker tests, the ability to target molecules, and ways of measuring and impacting the rate of aging. As a result of increased scientific interest, global private equity in the longevity space continues to grow at a rapid pace, supporting the work of doctors and scientists who are building this dynamic field, as well as other players in the longevity nation. "Elected officials and policymakers are also beginning to wake up and smell the demographics, looking at the financial insolvency of the Medicare and Social Security Trust Fund. They know they have to find answers," he said.[6]

Rowe is passionate about ensuring all the discoveries in the field become available to everyone, the democratization of healthcare being the important goal. "How do we make sure that the new drugs that can help to create longer, healthier lives become available and affordable to all people?" he asked, noting that having Medicare cover GLP-1 drugs would be a good example of delivering on this promise.[7]

Linda Fried

Dr. Linda Fried spent seventeen years as the dean and DeLamar Professor of Public Health, Mailman School of Public Health at Columbia University, as well as lecturing on the social capital of an aging society and on the assets and capabilities that we accrue with age. A geriatrician and epidemiologist, Fried now directs the Butler Columbia Aging Center, which includes the International Longevity Center USA, which

people are finally talking about healthy aging

focuses on global trends in healthy longevity and related policy responses.

In my conversation with Fried, she explained that people are finally talking about healthy aging.[8] Over the last thirty to forty years, public health science has provided evidence that health is malleable, she told me. "There's a recognition that building a society that invests in the assets of longer lives is a global agenda; accomplishing this would mean a lot to societies as well as individuals of all ages," she added.[9]

Along with Dr. John Eu-Li Wong, the Isabel Chan Professor in Medical Science and the senior vice president of Health Innovation and Translation at the National University of Singapore, Fried was cochair of the National Academy of Medicine's Global Roadmap for Healthy Longevity that was released in 2022. Joined by nineteen others, including Carstensen, Dr. Eric Verdin of the Buck Institute, and Drs. Jack Rowe and John Beard of Columbia, the ambitious report is a global call to action and a true road map. "It's a plan to put aging and longevity at the center of development agendas, an all-of-society plan with an intentional whole-of-society transformation," said Fried. "When the deputy prime minister of Singapore read it, he told us that he would be implementing the recommendations into their plan."[10]

According to Fried, the report is designed to improve physical, mental, and social well-being for people as they age. She noted that we live in a world that was designed when life expectancy was 47 versus nearly 80 or older in some countries today. As a result, the report focuses on the interconnectedness of social infrastructure, physical environment, health systems, and the longevity dividend, which is tapping into the knowledge and wisdom of older workers. For example, by working longer in life, older workers contribute more to GDP, pay more taxes, consume more, and contribute to intergenerational workforces, not to mention have better mental health and sense of purpose. Further, older people in the workforce lead to a stronger economy that creates more jobs for those who are younger.

Fried and her collaborators have working groups in Taiwan, South Korea, and China at ministerial levels, yet the group hasn't been able to find traction in the United States. She was part of New York Governor Hochul's State Master Plan for Aging and cochaired a subcommittee on Prevention and Healthy Aging, the first of its kind, with recommendations on state-based approaches to creating healthy longevity. But it has yet to lead to any substantive policy initiatives. There are currently twelve states with master plans on aging, but only New York State has included a focus on health promotion and disease prevention.

On the federal level, Fried believes that no congressperson over 50 would be caught talking about older people.[11] This creates inertia on the Hill, even as the demographic wave hits the United States with more than sixty million citizens currently 65 years or older.[12] As a global leader in public health, Fried is passionate about addressing healthy aging at the local, state, and federal levels and, more importantly, making programs available to all socioeconomic levels, particularly those with less access to healthcare.

Lynne Corner

In the United Kingdom, Lynne Corner is the chief operating officer at the National Innovation Centre for Ageing (NICA) at Newcastle University and director of Voice (Valuing Our Intellectual Capital and Experience).[13] Established fifteen years ago, Voice has a global network of tens of thousands of individuals who give input to businesses for products and services that are affordable, accessible, and relevant not just for an older population but for all people.

"The sharing of ideas that get people longevity ready might include architects designing lifetime homes or teachers creating new ideas for lifelong learning. The sharing of ideas from the members on our platform can help to improve design, product development, and more," said Corner.[14] One example is a project with Jaguar Land Rover UK, with member input on design for car buyers who are living longer and want certain kinds of features in their car choice.

The goal of NICA and Voice is to help businesses understand the enormous growth opportunities that are there due to people living longer and healthier lives. NICA was established in 2020, supported by an initial investment from the UK government and Newcastle University. Overseen by Director Nic Palmarini, the group is also focused on how AI can help to develop services and technologies for the longevity economy. A sister organization of NICA, Voice—with eight chapters in places like Italy, Germany, and Taiwan—is what Corner calls "the citizen voice at the heart of all that we do."[15]

Dan Buettner

Aside from the many experts in their fields who are building longevity nations, there is also a battalion of writers and social advocates who are helping people realize that the future is now. One such person is Dan Buettner, who sparked interest with his November 2005 cover story for *National Geographic*, "Secrets of Long Life." In the article, he identified five "blue zones," regions where people live long and healthy lives. According to Buettner, people in the blue zones have lower rates of chronic disease. They also have unique lifestyle factors like a plant-based diet and regular physical activity.[16] His passion for the subject has led to at least eight bestselling blue zone books with more on the way, as well as the Emmy Award-winning Netflix series *Live to 100: Secrets of the Blue Zones*.

When I spoke to Buettner, he had just completed his new book, *Blue Zones Kitchen: One Pot Meals*, which was published in the fall of 2025. When discussing the book, he said, "We want to get America eating healthier at home. Working with Stanford, we scraped 650,000 recipes, sorted them into five-star reviews, and then used an AI model to analyze them. We found seven flavor patterns that Americans love. We then hired the very best recipe developers, gave them the blue zone guidelines, and said that we want one-pot meals that take about a half an hour or less and cost under four dollars a serving."[17]

In addition, Buettner offers premade meals. Blue Zones Kitchen meals are frozen foods, as Buettner put it, "formulated for longevity and maniacally delicious."[18] Distributed in more than two thousand grocery stores, it's another way that his efforts are creating a healthier America. As he studied and researched the blue zones, Buettner applied many of the insights from those populations into the Blue Zones Project. Starting in 2009 in the town of Albert Lea, Minnesota, his pilot project was a community-wide initiative focused on improving health and well-being for better, longer lives.

"The program is now in seventy-five US cities with public support, but privately funded," he said, adding that "we let the public and private sectors evaluate each of the policies for effectiveness and feasibility in their city."[19]

The results have been impressive. Over a five-year period, the engaged communities saw drops in Body Mass Index (BMI) and reductions in heart disease, Type 2 diabetes, and even dementia, according to Buettner. When I asked him what one of his dream visions would be for the Blue Zones Project, he responded that he hoped the government would fund and support better health efforts for everyone.

As a thought leader in longevity, Buettner continues to remind everyone that many of the core fundamentals he has espoused continue to be the pathway to our own individual longevity (versus many of the fads and trends that have emerged in the longevity space). "I draw from human evolution and populations that have lived certain ways for centuries. They manifestly live longer, and they stand the test of time," he said.[20]

Paul Irving

Whenever I sit down with Paul Irving, it is always an intellectual feast. In so many ways, he is the ultimate Re-Imagineer role model of reinvention, and his breakthroughs have been in the longevity leadership space. After three decades in the national law firm

Manatt, Phelps & Phillips, many of them as chairman and CEO, he went on to a Harvard Advanced Leadership fellowship in his late 50s to explore what his next move might be. From there, he stepped into the role of president, then founder and chairman of the Center for the Future of Aging at the Milken Institute, and is now senior advisor at the institute. Add to that his long-time engagement with CoGenerate (a nonprofit committed to a world where older and younger people join forces to solve problems), his role as Distinguished Scholar in Residence at the USC Leonard Davis School of Gerontology, and his involvement in the Quadrivio Silver Economy Fund (one of the largest in the longevity investing space) and, well, you get the point about his broad set of interests. Now in his early 70s, Irving has spent fifteen years in the longevity sphere and has become an advocate and self-defined social scientist on the subject (including being a part of the National Academy of Medicine Global Commission on Healthy Aging and the 2015 White House Conference on Aging).

When I asked him if he has seen progress over his fifteen years in the longevity space, he said, "Yes, but it is still moving too slowly. Too many institutions still don't understand the challenges and opportunities that come with an aging society."[21]

Irving believes that private sector solutions will be much more important in a world where policy solutions are constrained. With the recent innovations in AI and technology, along with advances in bioscience, he sees a lot of potential. "There's a much brighter future for aging with these new developments. The advent of personalized aging with health and medicine will contribute to that, but so will interventions focused on lifelong learning and social connection, and intergenerational engagement," he said.[22] As an advocate for leaning into solutions for longer, better lives, Irving also espouses that "we need to get the message out

Too many institutions still don't understand the challenges and opportunities that come with an aging society

of the [academic] bubble of thought leaders and researchers into everyday policy, practice, media, and business."[23]

His successor at the Center for the Future of Aging at the Milken Institute is Managing Director Diane Ty, a long-established leader in the longevity space. She and her team of eight are focused on thought leadership in brain health, health span, home and community, and financial longevity, especially for caregiving and caregivers. "We want to reach investors, businesses, and policymakers on these topics to better inform them on what's happening in the world," she explained.[24]

The center conducts research, gathers consensus-based recommendations from multi-sector partners, and amplifies the findings to affect organizational practices and policies at the federal, state, and local levels. Some of their insights on brain health and home and community will be covered in later chapters.

Andrew Scott

I first became aware of Andrew Scott when I read *The 100-Year Life*, which he coauthored with Lynda Gratton, so when I met him during a trip to London, I was already a big fan of his work in the longevity sphere. A PhD from Oxford, he continues to have global influence on policymakers in how they adjust for the new longevity phenomenon. I have also been honored to speak to his class at the London Business School, where he is an economics professor, about how brands can grow their business by tapping into the new 50-and-up demographics with new products, marketing, and communication approaches.

Scott's book *The Longevity Imperative: How to Build a Healthier and More Productive Society to Support Our Longer Lives* is a call to action for building a better future, identifying the innovations needed in the economy and the financial sector as well as the health system.[25] One of the core prin-

a call to action for building a better future

ciples is his concept of the "evergreen economy" which harnesses the power of an aging population for economic growth and social good. As people live longer, it is a source of better productivity for societies and for individuals. "One of my goals with the book has been to get this topic on the agenda of politicians, policymakers, and businesses who can help to change the system," he said, adding that "governments are starting to wake up to the topic, the media is reporting on it, and there is a realization that finance, health, spiritual and personal issues are all interrelated in the longevity conversation."[26]

In 2024, Scott joined the Ellison Institute of Technology Oxford, where he is setting up his own Longevity Institute. His idea is to put money into hardcore research to find sustainable commercial solutions to stimulate the evergreen economy. "We want to create markets through alliances, finding out what works, spreading the word, and coming up with real ideas," he explained.[27]

His institute will focus on three topics that are central to longevity. The first two are economies that invest in the capacity of older people and healthcare systems that focus on keeping people healthier longer. One of the key questions Scott is focused on is whether we need a preventative health system for older people that is separate from the current health system. The third focus of the institute is identifying solutions that allow people to work longer, including skill building for career transitions. As he embarks on this new chapter, Scott will continue to be a Re-Imagineer in the longevity sector, a global voice for change in a time when living to 100 and older will be the norm.

"Aging" vs. "Longevity"

You may have noticed in this chapter that some organizations use the word aging and some use the word longevity. For example there's the Butler Columbia Aging Center and there's the Stanford Center on Longevity. At the University of Southern California there is the Longevity Institute and the Edward R. Royland Institute on Aging. The whole sector is in a state of transition with regard to its collective identity. Many would argue that longevity is a more positive word and brings more people into the conversation, even though aging and longevity are intertwined and interdependent on each other. As many have said, we start aging the day we are born, but we pursue healthy longevity throughout our lives.

There is an argument for both sides of the debate. Some would say call it what it is, but I'm advocating for *longevity* as the word that represents the collective work that is being done across the world. Using this term may even help destigmatize aging and the undercurrent of ageism that continues to exist in many cultures. After all, don't we all relate to the idea of a longevity nation versus an aging nation? That reframing underscores the work that this chapter's Re-Imagineer thought leaders have been doing on behalf of all of us.

The Re-Imagineers Going Forward

The Re-Imagineers I introduced in this chapter are but a fraction of the hundreds—maybe thousands—of leaders in the longevity space who are innovating in every sector and diligently working to create a longevity nation. While many of them have been at it for years, many more are just now joining in to build on the work of established Re-Imagineers. Their innovations will help millions flourish after middle age. But just as important are the countless everyday people who are living life to the fullest and acting as longevity role models. In the coming chapters, these Re-Imagineers will show us that a longevity lifestyle is available to everyone.

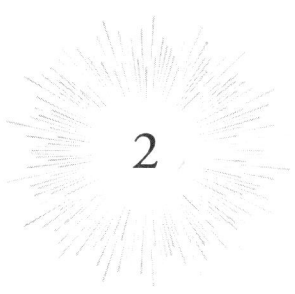

2

New Personas for a Longevity Nation

I n the first halves of our lives, our identities are often wrapped up in what I call the Three P's. We are focused on finding a life partner, becoming a parent (if that is one's choice), and starting some kind of profession or paying job to pay the bills. They are important identities, and they will be with us throughout our lives. However, they tend to evolve as we reach midlife.

For many of us, our child-rearing years are behind us once we reach our 50s. (Although, once a parent, always a parent. It's just that they need less from us as they become more involved in establishing their own lives.) But in a longevity nation, there are also those who are becoming first-time parents at 50 or older, and they are rearing children well into their 60s and beyond. If living to 100 is a possibility, this group may become first-time grandparents at 75 and even watch their grandchildren graduate from college.

If we partnered at 25, we may or may not have the same romantic relationship when we reach our 50s. Can we still find commonality with the same person twenty-five years later, or are we all destined for multiple partnerships throughout a longer life? A 2022 study revealed that 36 percent of US adults who divorced were over 50. Around 30 percent of Americans over 50 are single, including those who have never married as well as those who are divorced or widowed.[1]

Our 50s is usually the decade when we begin to wonder if we chose the right career path. After nearly thirty years in a profession, you might be burned out, disillusioned, frustrated, or just plain bored. Or your industry might have changed so much that you begin to think you need a change from it before they decide they need a change from you!

We all know how this can play out. The 60-year-old divorced person whose kids are gone gets downsized or laid off when their company is sold or reorganized. Suddenly, they're facing an identity crisis. I call it the midlife crisis 2.0.

Psychoanalyst Elliott Jaques coined the term "midlife crisis" in 1965.[2] With life expectancies of 70 years then, the "crisis" started earlier, oftentimes in the early 40s. With longer life expectancies, there is now a new existential moment when, at 60, we realize we may live another thirty years and need to rethink our identities. Finding new personas in the second half of life is something we all need to expect. It will help us live longer and happier lives. The question is, "what are your other P's?"

at 60, we realize we may live another thirty years and need to rethink our identities

In my book *ROAR: into the second half of your life (before it's too late)*, I introduced the concept of life layering in the chapter "Act Now with Life Layering," the most popular chapter in the book.[3] The idea is to build other identifiers or "personas" throughout life, so that our mental and emotional well-being isn't dependent on us fulfilling or adhering to a single, limited identity. These strong, lifelong personas can then sustain you for a lifetime. The book includes lots of tools and exercises to help you find your own path, as well as stories of people who found their way to new identities. Remember, what you do for a living is not who you are as a person. When you are done with a profession, it will always be a layer of your identity, but it's not one that you should linger on.

Perhaps the familiar example of someone who has failed to life layer is the guy who was the star quarterback in high school and twenty years later is still calling on that part of his life as his defining identity. It's the same with a CEO who steps down and becomes lost because they put all their self-worth and identity into that role. We all know that once you step out of that position, your life changes dramatically.

You can start the life-layering approach at any age, and the younger you start, the better you will be in terms of not putting all of your identity into the Three P's. I started life layering when I was 39 years old. Some of the new layers I built over the years include adventurer, photographer, writer, philanthropist, and marathon runner. I've baked this big layer cake of identities that now define me. My primary profession as a magazine publisher is still in me, but it is now secondary to how I define myself as a person.

Fortunately, there are people and organizations who are helping people become life-layering Re-Imagineers. Three key organizations in this space are the Modern Elder Academy, NxtWaves, and Camp Reinvention.

The Modern Elder Academy (M/E/A)

When I first started exploring the longevity phenomena, several people asked me if I knew Chip Conley. I'll admit that I didn't at the time, but finally I was able to have a coffee with him in Santa Fe, New Mexico. We have a family vacation home there, and Chip was there to build on his very successful midlife business. Let me just start by saying that Chip is a true force of nature. I immediately connected with his energy, vision, and enthusiasm. He is the founder of M/E/A, which stands for Modern Elder Academy, a school dedicated to helping people navigate midlife and beyond.[4] In Re-Imagineer parlance, M/E/A helps you build your new personas as you move into the future. At age 52, Chip began working at Airbnb, first as the head of global hospitality and strategy, then as strategic advisor for hospitality and leadership. It was at Airbnb that he became known as the "elder" advisor and helped grow the tech start-up into a global hospitality brand. In 2018, at the age of 58 (and developing another persona for himself), Chip launched M/E/A. Billed as the first midlife wisdom school, he established a campus in Baja, California, with life-changing workshops that help people in midlife find the clarity, purpose, and fulfillment they crave. A five-day workshop might include topics like identifying your situation and needs in the moment, or embracing the unknown as a pathway to possibility. In October 2025, I joined him at a new M/E/A campus outside of Santa

Fe to conduct a group session around life layering. More than seven thousand people from sixty countries have attended the workshops, led by leaders and experts from many different disciplines.

One of the alumni is Patrick McCleary. McCleary lives in Dallas, Texas, and followed a traditional career path that included an MBA and thirty years in the banking industry.[5] Then, when he was 55 years old, he started to realize he needed a change. Caring for his mother during her struggles with dementia and watching a 56-year-old friend deal with early-onset Alzheimer's and dementia was a bit of a wake-up call.

"I decided to step out and realized that I was a case study in burnout. At first, it was a lot of rest and reset, including yoga and Orangetheory," he said.[6]

After learning about M/E/A, McCleary signed up for a program at the Baja location about navigating transitions. What he learned during his time at M/E/A led to the creation of his newest persona: entrepreneur in the eldercare space. Using the tentative business name Act III—Eldercare, Estate & Transition Services, McCleary wants to create a concierge-like service that helps families and people plan their lives, including end of life. "As part of my learning, I'm also doing an eight-week online course at the University of Vermont called End-of-Life Doula Professional Certificate," he said.[7]

Don Spradlin is another graduate of the M/E/A programs. He first attended M/E/A in his early 70s and is now launching a new business in hospitality.[8] He spent a large part of his career in the non-profit world, as well as in the real estate business, but also became a Re-Imagineer in his 40s when he went back to school to earn a master's in clinical psychology to become a psychotherapist. "I did it for five years, but didn't like the rhythm of the one-on-one psychotherapy work, so I transitioned into doing organizational dynamics work," he said.[9]

Now a graduate of multiple M/E/A programs, Spradlin ultimately realized that one can be an entrepreneur at any age. In 2024, he launched a business called Joie de Vivre Homes that marries his deep experience in real estate with his love of travel. The business idea is to buy homes in Europe with a group of owners who will own shares in the house itself and have access to the home for multiple weeks throughout the year. Unlike the time-share model, this is ownership among individuals who like the idea of actually owning a piece of property but not taking on all the responsibilities

one can be an entrepreneur at any age

While large players like Ember and Pacaso have a similar model, Spradlin's goal is to be more bespoke, with a higher personal touch. At 77, he is excited about his new venture. When I asked him how long he might want to commit to the new business, he said, "When you get to be this age and be in good health and good spirits, you're damn lucky. I'd say I'll want to do this for another ten years."[10] Spradlin is part of the new breed of 70-somethings who still see that there is a lot they can accomplish.

Of course, McCleary and Spradlin wouldn't have benefited so completely from their time at M/E/A if it weren't for faculty members like Barbara Waxman. Waxman holds a master's degree in public administration and gerontology, and coaching certifications from the International Coach Federation and the Hudson Institute.[11] She is a sought-after longevity expert who has developed and taught multiple programs, including the Longevity Roadmap, a seven-module course that helps people chart a course toward becoming their new selves. "I'm focused on giving people a new life view," she explained.[12]

"We're living longer, but our systems, norms, and mindsets are still built for a younger, shorter-lived population. Many people don't yet realize the implications of this mismatch and need to take charge of their own well-being," she said.[13]

During the time he was assembling world-class Re-Imagineer leaders like Waxman, Conley was battling prostate cancer. He underwent surgeries, thirty-six successive daily radiation sessions, and eighteen months on hormone depletion therapy.[14] Throughout this long health journey, Chip has maintained a rigorous work schedule and continues to display passion and commitment to those who want to reinvent themselves in midlife.

NxtWaves

Another Re-Imagineer, Michele Evans, spent more than twenty-five years in HR leadership at Microsoft and Facebook/Meta, which included more than twelve years focusing on helping leaders grow. In her reimagined life, she launched NxtWaves, an organizational program for executives aiming for a meaningful post-corporate life and work. She has mentored hundreds of people who are ready to build their next chapter.[15] Her goal as a first-time entrepreneur was to help people transition into new chapters. Mark Buchanan was one of the people she helped. After an incredible twenty-two-year journey at Apple, he decided he wanted a change. An old boss told him that he was leaving a company with a strong culture and identity, and he would have to forge his own path.[16] The NxtWaves program helped him craft his new "Personal Purpose" plan identifying what he cared about. He decided on establishing a "portfolio life" of activities founded on the principles of the Japanese concept *ikigai*, which means "a reason to live."[17]

He identified seven activities for his new life's purpose, including focusing on his health and well-being, committing to helping leaders grow and evolve, becoming a life transition coach himself, and being the board cochair for Openhouse, a nonprofit that provides older LGBTQ+ adults safe, supportive housing, community programs, and services.[18] Now that he has found his own future path, Buchanan is always reminded of the quote from the late, great artist David Bowie, who said, "Ageing is an extraordinary process whereby you become the person you always should have been."[19]

Camp Reinvention

Dana Hilmer calls herself a midlife reinvention expert.[20] In early 2020, she and Wendy Perrotti, both trained coaches, cofounded and cofunded Camp Reinvention, the only program and community for women who dare to create a second half of their lives that they are wildly excited about. Several hundred women have gone through their various programs, including a twelve-week training program of reinvention that can be done online. Other offerings include immersive four-day retreats, the

Camp Reinvention Success Accelerators, and more. During a discussion in December 2024, Hilmer told me her group works with three different categories of women:

> One category is women who have checked a lot of boxes. They got married, had a family and a career. They've had a lot of success, but they are feeling a sense of emptiness. The second group is women who have put their life or dream on hold. They've been taking care of family, maybe elderly parents, and just haven't given themselves permission to actually be true to themselves and do what they really want. Our third group are women who have lost themselves and have no idea what they want anymore. They need to really get back to understanding who they are and what they want. The third group is a smaller subset of women whose lives haven't really worked out the way they had hoped. Maybe they were derailed by a loss of a career or a partner, a health crisis or that they never realized having a marriage and children. All of them come to us for these various reasons.[21]

Pamela Corante is an alum of Camp Reinvention. She has been a corporate communications officer for nearly thirty years, including stints at AT&T and the Motion Picture Association.[22] Committed to her career and lifelong learning, Corante also went through an MBA program at 50 as a way to enhance her professional journey.

"I had only experienced structured academic learning, so the idea of a form of coaching was not something I had considered. When I went to Camp Reinvention, I met a lot of women my age who were going through the same issues as me," she explained during a discussion I had with her in February 2025.[23] Through the program, Corante realized that she was on call for work 24/7, always ready for the next crisis. Therefore her life was, as she put it, "sucked of its joy."[24]

She made the commitment to spend more quality time with her husband and to make more room in her life for the things that she loved. One of those was re-enrolling in UCLA's creative writing program, as she has always dreamt of writing a novel. Camp Reinvention also reignited her desire to work for herself, something she had done already during her professional life: "We work so much, we should focus on doing the things that we really enjoy. While I was getting my MBA, I worked as a consultant and had a blast. It was the most fun I've ever had in a job."[25]

We work so much, we should focus on doing the things that we really enjoy

According to Corante, the exercises throughout the program led her to the question, "What's your guiding principle in life?" What do you want to shout from the rooftops when the meteor is about to hit. "My shout was I had a hell of a great time, and that forced me to realize that I wasn't really taking a lot of time in my life to enjoy what matters to me," she said.[26]

In her own ongoing reinvention, Hilmer has finished a retirement transition coaching program at the Retirement Coaches Association to expand the business that she has already built. "I would love to see companies change their mindset about retirement. There is an opportunity to look at their older workers in a different way, keeping them longer for mentoring, multigenerational work projects, and more, as they get on the road to leaving a career," she said.[27]

Embrace the Opportunity

As we discussed at the beginning of this chapter, our priorities shift as we age. While once we might have been fully focused on the Three P's, we now have the opportunity to explore new interests and layer our personalities in ways that benefit us and those around us. For some, that will mean taking part in innovative programs in non-academic settings, such as those offered by M/E/A, NxtWaves, and Camp Reinvention. For others, it may mean attending one of the new non-degree programs offered by schools like the University of Colorado at Denver, the Drucker School at Claremont University, or the University of Chicago. Still others may take a different route completely.

Regardless of the route they take, the point is that members of the longevity nation are embracing the midlife crisis 2.0 and realizing that they want to maintain a sense of purpose beyond the outdated retirement construct that says purpose and identity end in our 60s. As you now know, there is an array of organizations, companies, and institutions that are committed to helping anyone become a Re-Imagineer. So don't hesitate. The midlife crisis 2.0 is an opportunity to build new personas that will allow us all to expand beyond the identity of the Three P's as we live into our 90s or beyond.

members of the longevity nation are embracing the midlife crisis 2.0

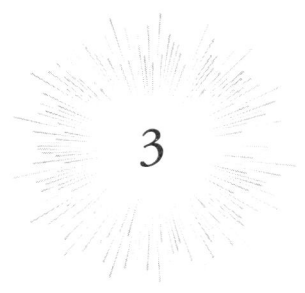

3

Lifelong Learning: Should You Go Back to School to Relaunch Your Life?

The aha moment of new longevity is realizing that we still have time, maybe decades, to pursue something different. As discussed in the previous chapter, that realization may lead you to enroll in a non-academic program to gain new skills and learn how to chart a new course for the rest of your life. What you learn may be enough to guide you to a new interest, a new purpose, or even a new business. But what if your first career choice didn't turn out to be what you thought it might be in terms of satisfaction, growth, and earning power? In that case, you have the opportunity to pursue an academic degree that builds on your years of experience in your current field or teaches you something completely new.

For example, Minnie Payne was a stay-at-home mom who sometimes worked as a transcriptionist and word processor. At 73, she went back to college at Texas Women's University to study journalism, leading her to copyediting and writing for various publications. When she was 90, she completed a master's degree in interdisciplinary studies from the University of North Texas, continuing to fine-tune her storytelling techniques.[1] Similarly, Guinness World Records identified Shigemi Hirata as the oldest college graduate in the world at age 96. At the age of 85, he enrolled in the Kyoto University of Art and Design in Kyoto, Japan. It took him eleven years to complete his ceramics studies there and receive his bachelor of arts degree.[2] Going back to school to expand on your craft like Minnie did or to pivot into a whole new world like Shigemi takes a personal commitment of your time and energy.

This raises the question: Should you go back to school to reboot? Or is pursuing a more informal form of education better for you?

Let's face it, by now your formal education, regardless of what you achieved or studied, has become totally obsolete. One thing we know is that the world around us is always changing, the most current example being the emergence of artificial intelligence. Think about how your own industry is changing. In my professional world, we went from being print-centric to all forms of digital, including websites, social media, video, e-commerce, and now artificial intelligence and personalization.

If you have come to the realization that it is your time to strike out in a new way, read my friend Avivah Wittenberg-Cox's essay in *Forbes* called "Aging Relevantly: Getting Good at Midlife Transitions." In the article, she explains how we have to learn to let go of our first-half-of-life achievement goals, tackle the messy middle when you are trying to figure out what's next, and embrace the new beginnings, or who you will become in the second half of life.[3]

Aside from your own motivation and interest, the two biggest questions that come up on this subject is how does one find the time and where does one find the money. Let's talk about finding the time. (There's a lot of money available for people over 40 who want to go back to school, a topic that we'll cover later in this chapter.)

Finding the Time

Time is yours to control, and we all know how and where we can edit out the wasted hours in our lives to fill them with more engaging and meaningful pursuits. I learned this myself when I realized that I was spending countless hours scrolling through social media platforms. What was I really accomplishing during all that time? In the end, I realized it was like junk food: It added no value to my life. Instead, I used that time in more purposeful ways, like reading a book on a subject that interested me.

President Teddy Roosevelt was a master at finding the time to pursue multiple activities. Not only did he rise to the position of president, but he authored eighteen books, helped raise six children, and was a committed conservationist. He established 150 National Parks and saved 230 million acres of American wilderness.[4] Even as he suffered through the deaths of his wife and his mother, who both died on the same day, he persevered to accomplish an enormous amount in his life. In his speech "The Strenuous Life," he argued that strenuous effort and overcoming hardship was better for individuals

I was spending countless hours scrolling through social media platforms

and the country.[5] If you don't think you have enough time to go back to school to learn something new, read up on Teddy for your inspiration.

If his story doesn't help you, then turn to some everyday individuals who have made it a priority to move it forward on the educational front.

One of my favorite stories is Anh Vu Sawyer's personal journey. She and her family were evacuated from Vietnam during the fall of Saigon. They lived in five refugee camps before landing in Oakbrook, Illinois, where a Christian Reform church helped them find their footing in America. Sawyer went to college in the United States, married, and had children. She worked in the nonprofit sector, including ten years as executive director of the Southeast Asian Coalition of Central Massachusetts, where she led the organization's mission to support immigrants, refugees, and low-income residents. After nearly four decades of juggling full-time work and raising a family, she said that "something happened" in her early 60s. "Because of all of my family responsibilities, like many women, I put aside my own big dreams," she said in a profile in OprahDaily.com. "Now that the kids were independent and all out of college, I was ready to pursue those dreams with abandon."[6]

While continuing to work full time, she also tutored immigrant kids in high school. She made a deal that if they applied to college, she would apply to a graduate program. All twenty of her students applied to college, and all of them were accepted. Sawyer decided to apply for an MBA at Massachusetts Institute of Technology and was accepted at age 66. She was ready to start her Re-Imagineer journey. As she explained in the OprahDaily article, she had no idea how she was going to pay for it, as she and her husband didn't have a lot of money. "I almost had to sell our house twice and ultimately refinanced, but I found a scholarship," she said.[7]

When some of her fellow students learned about her financial situation, they helped raise money to complete her tuition payments. Not only did she graduate from MIT, but then she went on to the one-year Harvard Advanced Leadership Initiative on a full scholarship. At nearly 70, Sawyer launched her entrepreneurial business with the help of a grant from the Massachusetts Growth Capital Corporation and other sources. Next, she wants to build a business that has a positive social impact. Her plan is to engage immigrant and refugee communities in producing a line of sustainable clothing for women over 40 that's both affordable and stylish.[8]

David Harrison is another career Re-Imagineer who pursued an education in a new field while continuing to work in his current profession. As a United Airlines international first officer pilot on the 787 Dreamliner aircraft, he is required to retire at 65. While there have been recent attempts to extend the retirement age to 67, so far they have not succeeded, although pilots can fly beyond age 65 in non-commercial environments.[9]

To get ready for his next chapter, Harrison enrolled in Columbia University's Wealth Management program. The decision was sparked by the death of an important father figure and mentor. Harrison watched as his friend's final wishes were not honored, and he became interested in the idea of estate management.

His sixteen-month asynchronous program, with residencies at the beginning and at the end, allows him to continue working as a pilot as he sets himself up for his new career. Harrison wants to honor his mentor's legacy by bringing the work ethic, humility, integrity, and principles the man embodied into the field of wealth management. Whether it involves complex estate planning, managing liquidity events, or simply introducing a 9-year-old to the concept of compounding interest from her lemonade stand profits, he is getting ready for what could be another thirty-year career.

New Models of Higher Education

The world of higher education has created incredible new education models for those who want to pursue new studies. Universities have to think in more innovative ways, as their traditional model is facing significant challenges like "the demographic cliff." According to *Inside Higher Ed*, given declining birth rates over the last decade, the number of 18-to-24-year-olds in the United States "will peak in 2025 and then decline dramatically for several years."[10] In a double hit, the number of 18-to-24-year-olds choosing to attend college has been in decline for several years due to changing attitudes about education and the rising cost of a college degree.

However, there is an enormous opportunity for universities to focus on the midcareer professional who wants to either build on their expertise or pivot in a new direction. It's already happening across the board. The growth of Schools of Professional Studies, certificate programs, online degrees and year-long programs for post-career lives are all thriving. Schools of Professional Studies (SPS) can be found around the country at places like the University of North Carolina in Charlotte, the University of Central Missouri, Salem State, and New York University. At NYU's SPS, you can earn an undergraduate or master's degree but also get a continuing education certificate in emerging industries if you're pursuing career change or advancement. Some subjects include AI and emerging technology, electrical, HVAC, plumbing, project management, and cannabis.

Universities have to think in more innovative ways

Alternatively, you may decide that a career in the new longevity sector is appealing to you. There are lots of established and new programs emerging, including the University of Southern California's online part- or full-time master's degree in nutrition, healthspan, and longevity. The University of Florida offers a master's degree in innovative aging studies. In Europe, there are similar programs at the University of Pavia in Italy and at the Geneva College of Longevity Science in Switzerland, which offers an executive master in longevity science.

When I visited the National University of Singapore (NUS), I learned from Dr. Andrea Maier and her colleague Louis Island that they have introduced new learning modules for those who want to expand their training and knowledge. The Academy for Healthy Longevity is part of the Yong Loo Lin School of Medicine there, offering diverse courses and programs designed to prepare people at all levels to excel in the emerging field of geroscience and healthy longevity. For example, young professionals can take advantage of NUS's twelve-day Healthy Longevity Talent Incubator program, while established health-care professionals may choose to join the Healthy Longevity Intensive Course. In addition, they plan to begin offering a new master's degree in healthy longevity in 2026.[11]

My own story fits into this narrative. I've always considered myself a lifelong learner. I thrived in college, studying economics and political science as an undergraduate and then earning an MBA in marketing. I loved everything about school and how it stretched my knowledge base.

The philanthropy world has always been one of my deep interests, as I have served on many nonprofit boards. While it was never my plan to move into a full-time role of president or executive director of a non-profit organization, it was my goal to learn as much as I could about the sector so that it would make me a better board member and philanthropist. I wanted to learn about new forms of fundraising, change management, and legal and tax issues, and gain an overall understanding of how different parts of the nonprofit world operated and how it was being disrupted by technology. In 2021, I earned my master of science degree in nonprofit management at Columbia University. My brain was filled with an incredible amount of knowledge that I put to work in all of my philanthropic endeavors. During the process, I also developed an amazing cadre of friends, including my fellow "midlife" student, Donna Emma, a former Wall Streeter who was moving into a new career chapter as cochair of the Massachusetts General Hospital Leadership Council for Psychiatry.

My friend Jeanne Marin also decided to pursue a midlife career change. She was already a highly recognized dermatologist and surgeon, but in her mid-50s she went back to school to become a veterinarian. When I asked her about her experiences, she told me, "The most difficult aspect was not necessarily the complexity or volume of material, but the acute and severe change in my life. There were days that I was disheartened, and then there were days of pure joy. I remained determined."[12]

According to Marin, veterinary school was infinitely more demanding than medical school had been. Human doctors only have one species to master, while veterinarians study many species, each with their own anatomy, physiology, disease states, and more. "I enjoyed the interactions with students half my age, and the special friendships that I made. I enjoyed academic success and exceeding everyone's expectations of an older student. If you asked me 'Would you do it again?' the answer is a definitive yes," she said.[13]

There were days that I was disheartened, and then there were days of pure joy

Now, at 60, Marin is embarking on a new career. When we spoke in the spring of 2025, she explained that she is still a novice, but her new work colleagues have been kind and nurturing and have helped her thrive. Her goal is to improve the lives of animals. She finds joy in her daily contributions as she builds her new profession. She also continues to dream of making a bigger impact on the national and global level over time.

University-Affiliated Alternative Academic Programs

While going back to college for an undergraduate, graduate, or doctoral program may not be your thing, you can still take on a meaningful experience in the academic world to put your brain to work. There are different programs, certificates, short courses, and more that can put you on your Re-Imagineer course.

Kate Schaefers has a PhD in counseling psychology from Iowa State University and has been an academic Re-Imagineer in higher education for most of her adult life. Currently director of the Osher Lifelong Learning Institute at the University of Minnesota, she also ran the university's Advanced Careers Initiative and spearheaded the 2025 launch of the Midlife Academy.

Schaefers is also the colead of the Nexel Collaborative with Simon Chan, a Canadian thought leader in longevity. The Collaborative officially started at Stanford under a grant from the Hewlett Foundation in 2018. It became an independent nonprofit entity under the fiscal sponsorship of Community Initiatives. Twenty-seven colleges and universities around the world are members, sixteen of which have active programs (or soon to be launched), plus eight individual advocate members. The institutional members provide midlife transition programs that help midlife students find new purpose and meaning, make new social connections, and engage across generations. The goal is to have programs for people of all levels. And while some of the institutions are more expensive than others, most of them have financial aid and scholarships for eligible students.[14]

The University of Chicago's Leadership and Society Initiative (LSI) is an example of another program designed to help accomplished leaders live meaningful lives by activating their encore chapters for the good of society. (For full disclosure, I'm on the advisory board of LSI.) According to Seth Green, dean of the Graham School of Continuing Liberal and Professional Studies at the University of Chicago, people typically join the LSI Fellowship within a year of finishing a seminal chapter in their careers.[15] The end of a longstanding career, then, requires reimagining your relationships, identity, impact, and learning agenda.

"LSI's curriculum starts with a course, taught jointly by faculty from the university's Booth School of Business and the humanities division, where the students, or "fellows," contemplate their core values by reflecting on their life experiences and reading timeless philosophical texts," explained Green.[16]

The end of a longstanding career, then, requires reimagining your relationships, identity, impact, and learning agenda

Ultimately, a fellow develops a "Purpose Plan" that helps them set the course for their reimagined future. In addition, the University has added a second pathway called Crafting Your Next Chapter. The program includes a class that meets virtually every other Tuesday for two hours and includes goal-setting and individual coaching.

The University of Colorado, Denver, has a similar program called Change Makers. Started in 2023, the program culminates in participants writing a ninety-day plan on how to transition into a next job, wind down a career, or find another purpose.[17]

Marc Freedman, the founder and co-CEO of CoGenerate, an organization committed to bridging generational divides to create the future, is also founding faculty codirector of the Yale Experienced Leaders Initiative (ELI).[18] Launched in 2025, this program is designed for working adults who may not be able to commit to spending a full year on campus. "Our goal is to create a six-month program that is a week on campus for the first week and a return to campus for the last week. We see this as a newly emerging kind of curriculum for individuals who want to get on a path to finding their next purpose," he explained.[19]

The programs that offer coursework to help you reimagine your next chapter are limitless. It's just a matter of identifying what it is you want to do.

Jane Lodato held senior marketing roles in Hollywood and the tech and finance industries before reimagining her life in her 60s and becoming a certified mindfulness teacher. To acquire the skills she needed to teach, mentor, and coach, she attended a rigorous training program sponsored by UC Berkeley's Greater Good Science Center. Later, when she met the chair of surgery for the Mount Sinai Hospital System at an event, she asked if mindfulness was part of the curriculum or was offered to the surgeons. It led to a deeper conversation, which then led to Lodato relocating from the Bay Area to New York City as she approached 70. Her new chapter was launched.[20]

At Católica University in Lisbon, Portugal, the innovative Longevity Leadership Program is the first of its kind. Designed for leaders in both public and private sectors, the program prepares participants for the economic, social, and workplace impacts of the world's new demographic reality and fast-aging societies. Developed by Avivah Wittenberg-Cox, longevity expert, and Professor Celine Abecassis-Moedas, the weeklong program attracts leaders from across the world: like César Garcia, a silver economy specialist at IFC World Bank in Mexico City, and Mafalda Hónorio, the head of longevity marketing at Fidelidade, the global insurance company.[21]

"Longevity will increasingly be on a par with issues like climate change and artificial intelligence," said Abecassis-Moedas, underscoring why a career in the space will be more and more relevant.[22]

Regardless of your career stage, helping your company and industry get longevity ready is an exciting new concept. It will also open a new dimension for business leadership. "Addressing longevity is no longer optional; it is a strategic imperative for businesses seeking resilience and growth in the decades to come," said Wittenberg-Cox.[23]

Although these alternative academic programs generally take less time to complete than a typical bachelor's degree, they still require considerable commitment. If you are looking for a first step into an academic setting before charting a new yearlong-or-more program, you may want to explore the Osher Lifelong Learning Institutes, which operate on the campuses of 125 institutions of higher education across the country. Their non-credit courses are designed for people 50 and older who love the joy of learning.

Paying for School

Now that you have learned about all the academic paths you might take to create your own Re-Imagineer story, there is still that lingering question about how you will pay for it? Programs can range from less than $500 (the Osher Lifelong Learning Institute) to more than $70,000 for the Harvard Advanced Leadership Initiative. But there is a lot of money that is available if you take the time, do the research, and hone in on what might be most relevant for you.

take the time, do the research, and hone in on what might be most relevant for you

In a ChatGPT search of "financial resources for people over 40 who want to go back to school," six meaningful answers came up. The FAFSA is the Free Application for Federal Student Aid. There are also Pell Grants, the Federal Supplemental Education Opportunity Grant (FSEOG), ScholarshipsandGrants.us, LendingTree's Scholarship Guide, and the Federal Student Aid Toolkit. There are many private scholarship funds too. They include the Ford Opportunity Scholarship, the Imagine

America Adult Skills Education Program, and the Jeannette Rankin scholarship, which is geared toward women 35 and up in technical or vocational education.

If you hit a roadblock in finding financial aid or don't want to dip into your own savings, there is still a path to be a Re-Imagineer for little or no cost. Coursera and edX are good sources to explore, as is the OpenLearn platform from Open University, United Kingdom. The Indian Institute of Technology offers free online courses. If you are intentional about your search, you'll also find free courses at prestigious schools like MIT's OpenCourseWare and Open Yale Courses at Yale University.

Limitless Opportunities

The opportunities for lifelong learning are available at every level you can imagine. If your goal is to reskill, upskill, learn something new, or expand on what you know already, this chapter was written not only to inspire you on what is out there, but also to share some of the incredible Re-Imagineer stories of the people who are leading the charge and those who have already done the work.

In the longevity era, revisiting education at any age to launch a new career or just to be a lifelong learner is not only good for your knowledge gain, but also for your brain health. If you are looking for a growth industry that will allow you to flourish at any age, moving into the longevity sector is a great option. You will become one of the architects of longevity nation and help determine what it will mean for millions now and in the future.

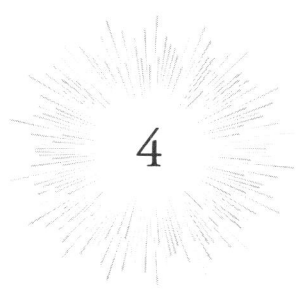

4

Workplaces Reimagined
for Longer Lifespans

Across the globe, the business world is facing a daunting challenge. Their rapidly aging workforce is creating a significant talent drain that may stall productivity, hamper growth prospects, and force a complete rethink on retaining, retraining, and promoting their over-50 talent. In addition, the global workforce is already the oldest in history and will continue to age. A Bain & Company study projected that by 2030, 150 million jobs worldwide will have shifted to workers over 55. (That's almost equivalent to the entire US workforce.)[1] If a company wants to maintain talent and performance, it will require reimagining work models and benefits, as well as focused attention on what these workers want and need.

"Companies don't have an option," said Michele Evans.[2] Evans spent twenty-five years in executive HR roles at Microsoft and Meta and is the founder and CEO of NxtWaves, a membership group that promotes long-term career vibrancy. "The talent gap is real, and planning for it over the next decade or so will give them a true competitive advantage."[3]

As millions of baby boomers around the world leave their jobs, there aren't enough people in the next generation to fill the void. Add in that the first millennials turn 50 in the year 2031, and it becomes obvious that employers will need to think of new ways to engage their 50-plus-year-old employees. It's also a long-term trend, as fewer babies are being born around the world, particularly in developed countries.

According to a study from the McKinsey Global Institute, two-thirds of humanity lives in countries where the birth rate is lower than the replacement level of 2.1 children per family, meaning populations will continue to shrink. By 2100, populations in some major areas will have fallen by 20–50 percent.[4] Having fewer working-age people will result in slower growth in hours worked and thus reduce GDP per capita growth, not to mention straining state pensions and Social Security. While it is true that AI may relieve some of the pressures, there's no guarantee that this is any type of magic bullet to solve the issue. However, there are a number of things that companies and other organizations can do during this workplace revolution to preserve the unique skills of older employees.

Creating an Age-Inclusive Culture

As people live longer, their capacity and desire to work longer increase, whether they want the income or the sense of purpose or both. This presents a big opportunity for businesses, but many fail to take advantage of it. Instead, even as healthy people in their mid-50s begin to realize that they may live into their 90s, many of them are discovering that their employers are more focused on moving them out of the workplace than on finding ways to keep them. This attitude on the part of businesses is a structural issue that was created at a time when life expectancies were much lower. Unfortunately, the business world has been slow to recognize this as a major issue that no longer serves employees or employers. However, there are Re-Imagineers who are working to spread awareness of this issue and make it a matter of urgency for everyone.

employers are more focused on moving them out of the workplace than on finding ways to keep them

Mike Mansfield is the CEO of ProAge .org, a UK-based charity whose mission is to equip business leaders with the intelligence to create an age-inclusive culture. "We did a survey of 225 organizations to see how they were preparing for the demographic change of an aging workforce. Using a scale of 1 to 10, the average answer was 7.2 for acknowledging that it is an important topic, but the answer was only 4.2 for how strategically prepared they were to act on it," he said.[5]

His group works with major companies like Coca-Cola Euro Pacific Partners, using awareness training programs and practical solutions to come up with ways to attract and retain older workers. The conversations also include how government policy might help employers. "Invariably someone says a tax incentive would help," he said.[6]

It's not an unusual idea. Sweden, Germany, and Canada all have incentives in place. As of 2025, even the United States has a federal program called Work Opportunity Tax Credit (WOTC) that offers tax credits for hiring within specific groups, including older workers facing employment challenges. The Organisation for Economic Co-operation and Development (OECD) has a report called the Council Recommendation on Ageing and Employment Policies that includes other ideas for companies to create a more age-inclusive commitment.

As businesses begin adapting to the aging workplace, Mansfield sees new kinds of initiatives emerging: Multi-generational resource groups create natural engagement among generations. Some companies offer menopause services as benefits. Under the Apprenticeship Levy, the UK government funds 95 percent of the training for all age groups, including mid-career professionals who want to upskill or change careers.[7]

Going forward, everyone will be thinking about having a sixty-year career to fund a 100-year life. Building a workplace infrastructure to support this dimension for a longevity nation should be top of mind for all business leaders, especially since the idea of a linear career in a company or industry is already becoming less appealing to younger generations. For someone who follows Stanford's New Map of Life road map, that will mean a lifetime series of career breaks followed by reentry to the workforce, with constant reskilling and upskilling to remain relevant. If a company wants to retain talent, they'll need to adjust to this new reality.

Reskilling and Upskilling

Mitchell Stevens, a professor of education and sociology at Stanford and a big thinker on the topic of reskilling and upskilling, is spearheading an initiative called the Futures Project. He and his colleagues are working on building a national vision for human capital in the future with the report *Building a Learning Society*. With the rapid changes in work and technology, he advocates for a new approach, saying, "We need to shift from an education mindset to a learning mentality. As we all live longer lives, we need to build in reskilling and upskilling throughout an employee's entire work lifespan."[8]

This reimagining of how employers and individuals can keep pace with change will require new thinking and investment from government, companies, and employers. The need for ongoing skills training is no longer a "nice to have" but will be critical for building an environment of what Stevens calls "lifelong employability."[9]

However, this mindset shift on the part of employers won't be instantaneous. In the meantime, Kerry Hannon, the author of fourteen books, including *In Control at 50+: How to Succeed in the New World of Work*, believes it is up to the individual to have a lifelong learning mindset with regard to obtaining new skills. "Raise your hand and ask for it. You cannot be passive in today's workplace. If you want to keep working, you have to make sure that you are staying on top of new kinds of skills."[10]

As a workplace futurist, she is always looking for new models of the future, which might include transitioning to part-time work or post-career engagements between employers and employees. She cites Michelin as a best-practice company that is one step ahead in helping its employees continue to learn and grow, regardless of their age: "An employee is assigned a career coach that tracks them throughout their time at Michelin. As they age, they may shift to different departments and areas during their time there."[11]

Michelin has four hundred dedicated career managers who work with employees to understand their interests and passions.[12] There is an ongoing skills enhancement program, and employees can try new career paths. This ensures employee retention. According to Hannon, as employees wind down their careers, Michelin uses them to represent the company in the community.[13] They also have a very active retiree group that they bring back to do all kinds of things. With a goal to retain, retrain, and tap into the knowledge and experience of their employees, the Michelin model is already one step ahead in keeping employees engaged longer.

Hannon also believes there is a big opportunity for companies and institutions of higher education to collaborate on reskilling. Cuyahoga Community College (Tri-C) in Cleveland, Ohio, is a great example. They operate a Mobile Training Unit that goes to companies, community events, and other venues to promote manufacturing and training for the next generation of workers, as well as upgrade skills and improve processes for current workers. Keeping pace with the region's manufacturing skills needs, the training programs include welding techniques, 3D printing, and programmable logic control.

There are other thought leaders, consultants, practitioners, and innovative companies who are focused on ideas and solutions for a longevity nation. For example, Lyndsey Simpson is the founder of the UK-based 55/Redefined Group, a firm that enables companies to retain, retrain, and hire talent over 50.[14]

Simpson told me about a global investment bank client who informed her they weren't really concerned about the risks of an aging workforce: "When I asked them to share their employee profile, it was 2 percent boomers, 27 percent Gen X, and 67 percent millennial. When I made them realize that in four years, they would have a significant shift into a 50-plus-year-old employee profile with their millennial base, you should have seen the fireworks in the room."[15]

According to a Pew Research study, the older workforce in America has nearly quadrupled in size since the mid-1980s, and the US Bureau of Labor Statistics predicts that older adults will account for 57 percent of labor force growth over the next decade. People 75 and older are the fastest-growing age group in the workforce.[16] On a global scale, 40 percent of the working-age population in OECD countries is made of people age 45–64, a significant increase from 28 percent in 1990.[17]

older adults will account for 57 percent of labor force growth over the next decade

How will companies adapt to this changing employee profile and avoid the talent drain?

According to Simpson, the dismissive approach to the needs of older workers is not uncommon. She revealed that in an aggregation of the data of users of her company's platform, regarding employees 50 and over, 93 percent of those surveyed reported that their employers did not provide them with any support.[18]

In the United States alone, 10,000 people a day are turning 65,[19] and while many of them are opting for a traditional retirement, the new breed of Re-Imagineers view retirement as an outdated concept. They see themselves as healthy, motivated, and ambitious. Their goals are to learn more, continue to contribute, and earn income. If they cannot do it at their current company, they are looking for other places to work, taking their experience with them. Or they are starting new careers at 65 with the potential of another ten to twenty years of work that excites them.

One example is Jeanne Noonan, who spent thirty years in the media business but decided it was time to embark on a new career. "My job was no longer creative or fun. I wasn't happy, and it was time to take stock about what I wanted to do next. When I thought about what I was passionate about, it was interior design, as my job exposed me to working with the best designers in the country."[20] Noonan applied to the New York School of Interior Design and landed a job with an NYC-based architecture and design firm. "I'm opening myself up to what I don't know, learning quickly, and becoming a valuable member of our team," she said.[21]

As we've discussed throughout this chapter, the risk for many companies is that if they do not accommodate the needs of experienced employees, they will lose their knowledge and insights.

Simon Chan is a Canada-based longevity and future of work, learning, and retirement strategist in the financial services sector and higher education. He sees countless examples of how businesses are affected by talent drain. "When I talked to the Chief Technology Officer of a big pension plan client, he told me that due to so many people retiring, they ran out of people who actually understood their technology systems. They had to go to their retirees and brought a few of them back to work on the system but also become a mentor to someone who could work within the system," he explained when I spoke with him in February 2025.[22]

This new model of "returnships" is one way companies can tap into expertise: A company rehires a former employee who has deep knowledge, skills, and experience that can help the company achieve its goals. But according to Chan, there are no real institutional systems in place to address the issue. "There's no sense of urgency with many business leaders on this topic. A lot of it is negotiated on an individual basis. Companies need better approaches for their aging workforce."[23] One of his clients is introducing a new kind of employee workshop that helps off-ramp an employee who is leaving the company. It's beneficial for both the employee and the employer, but it's obviously of limited use to employees who wish to continue working.

It's time to reframe work for employees over 50 and abolish the idea that 65 is an end date in one's career. Smart employers are realizing they need to keep experienced, long-term players by rethinking their role in their employee base. Those who do this also open themselves up to the possibility of retaining the skills of older workers even after those workers decide they are ready to leave the workforce.

> **Smart employers are realizing they need to keep experienced, long-term players**

Using AI to Transfer Skills

It has long been a tradition for older, more experienced workers to pass along their skills and knowledge to newer, less experienced workers. However, a variety of factors can limit the effectiveness of the knowledge transfer. For example, the older employee may leave the firm before their replacement can be identified, or there may be a mismatch between teaching and learning styles. However, the advent of AI opens up new possibilities when it comes to preserving the skills of older workers for the long term.

Kevin Delaney is the cofounder, CEO, and editor in chief of Charter, a future-of-work media and research company, and he believes that some dominant workplace trends, such as the increasing role of AI, may be favorable for an aging workforce.[24]

"If older workers engage with learning AI technology, there's a special opportunity for them. With their years of experience, they can become AI agents, managing the work on AI within an organization. That includes identifying the types of skills needed, assessing the work, giving feedback, and improving on it," he said.[25] Using AI tools to transfer knowledge between older and younger employees also allows for wisdom to be shared across generations as a new kind of mentoring.

Efforts to Avoid Talent Drain Around the World

Aside from France, where the legal retirement age is 64, many developed countries around the world are setting the retirement age at 67, depending on someone's year of birth. These are the ages when Social Security or state pensions can be fully realized. However, each nation has a slightly different approach to the topic of retirement.

For example, in the United Kingdom, it's illegal for a company to have a mandatory retirement age. However, the age one can start receiving state pension is rising to 67 between 2026 and 2028, depending on an individual's birthdate.[26] In Denmark, full public pension currently starts at 66, but they are already thinking about how to recalibrate their system based on their citizens living longer lives.[27] Starting in 2030, the government will set the retirement age based on life expectancy figures and adjust its pension plan accordingly. By 2040, the Danish retirement age will be 70 for those born after December 31, 1970.[28]

Many think that official retirement ages will continue to move into the late 60s or early 70s as governments realize that their systems are not sustainable because the number of people drawing state funds is much higher than those paying into it. How are companies beginning to shift their thinking due to these huge demographic changes?

One of the best initiatives is happening in France, where a group of CEO Re-Imagineers has started to map out a new kind of work environment and updated policies for the longevity era. Currently, 64 percent of working French people believe that being over 50 is a barrier to employment, even when one's skills are equal to younger candidates.

And yet by 2030, more than 30 percent of France's population will be over 60.[29] To combat age-based discrimination in the workplace, 136 French companies as diverse as Air France, L'Oréal, and AXA have signed a charter, initiated by Club Landoy, to retain, retrain, promote, and hire employees 50 and older.

In the *Forbes* article "CEOs Get Serious About Longevity Leadership—in France," Sibylle Le Maire, president of Club Landoy, states, "The issue is not to ask people to work longer but to give them better opportunities. The demographic transition requires a new social pact and a reevaluation of work itself."[30] Written by longevity expert Avivah

The issue is not to ask people to work longer but to give them better opportunities

Wittenberg-Cox, the article outlines four KPIs to measure a company's starting point and evaluate the process over time. They include the number of 50-and-older employees, training hours spent on them versus younger employees, recruitment rates for 45-and-older employees, and job mobility metrics for older employees. The companies that sign the charter agree to ten commitments, which are designed to combat ageism and develop and invest in employees over 50.

L'Oréal has taken the commitment globally in an effort called the For All Generations program. With more than fifteen thousand employees over 50, the company is deeply committed to supporting their employees through a long career journey. The five pillars of the program include promoting intergenerational diversity to change the perception of experienced employees; adapting health and well-being initiatives at work, such as Menopause Day; developing employability throughout one's career, including upskilling; facilitating a successful transition to retirement when that day comes; and facilitating new life projects post-L'Oréal.[31] In the United States, the L'Oréal for All Generations Program is a thriving part of the company's culture. "In this new environment, where age inclusivity will be vital, we must not only recruit and develop talent at all stages of their careers with well-being benefits to match, but . . . create opportunities for people to exchange their valuable knowledge and experiences with enthusiasm. As someone who has been building a career for nearly 40 years, I personally welcome this evolution," said David Greenberg, CEO of L'Oréal USA and president of the company's North America Zone.[32]

The United Kingdom has a similar commitment with the Age-Friendly Employer Pledge to foster age-inclusive workplaces for individuals over 50. The Certified Age Friendly Employer (CAFE) program in the United States is another example, as is the Later Life Workplace Index (LLWI) in Germany.

While all of these are great efforts, real policies and practical solutions have to be embedded into the everyday activity of the company.

Integrating Age-Inclusive Reforms into Company Culture

In the United States, CVS Health, Microsoft, and Marriott are often cited as companies that have done the work to make changes. Microsoft, for example, made age-inclusive reforms that include health coverage without employee premiums, caregiver leave, and maintaining benefits for employees who move from full-time to part-time.[33]

There are lots of emerging suggestions for employers to lean into their midcareer employees with better benefit offerings that are relevant to their stage of life. For example, in the *Harvard Business Review* story "How Companies Can Support Employees Experiencing Menopause," Bradley Schurman and Tamsen Fadal discuss ways to support midcareer female employees, advocating for ideas such as extending benefits for menopause support, holding company events on the topic, and listening to employees through surveys, among other approaches.[34]

Individually, Schurman and Fadal are both active in the longevity space. Schurman, the author of *The Super Age: Decoding Our Demographic Destiny*, is also the founder of Human Change, tracking important trends around the world connected to demographic insights. Fadal, a former television anchor, wrote her own bestselling book *How to Menopause* in 2025 and has become a global leader in helping companies recognize the importance of supporting their female employees during this time of their lives. The book provides practical advice and strategies from a team of more than forty experts, including doctors and therapists, to help women navigate menopause.

Yvonne Sonsino is the former total well-being and longevity lead at Mercer, the global consulting firm that specializes in human resources. She helped companies get a better understanding of how to keep their over-50 employees in the workforce longer.[35]

In 2024, Mercer conducted a survey in which it asked its clients about their efforts to support employees over 50. The survey revealed that companies are developing programs to support employee well-being, such as later-life health screenings and training in financial literacy, especially for women. "There is a gender pension gap between men and women that can be up to 40 percent in developed countries. Since women live six to seven years more than men, it's a real issue," Sonsino explained when we spoke in March 2025.[36] One of the key findings of the survey is that about 65 percent of older employees value flexibility, so many companies are working to give employees the opportunity to shape their own hours or work from home.

Unilever developed a new approach to flexibility with their U-Work program after realizing that almost a third of their UK workforce was eligible for retirement within the next five years.[37] According to the *Forbes* article "Flexibility for All: Unilever's Vision of the Future of Work," employees who opt in to U-Work have a contract rather than a traditional job. They get a guaranteed minimum monthly retainer representing a portion of their former salary, with some additional benefits like healthcare and pension contributions. Then they're additionally paid per project, choosing how long and how often to work. Older employees might tap into the program differently than younger employees choose to, but all age groups appreciate the flexibility. It can also work as a way to transfer skills to the next generation, particularly when an individual identifies it's time to start planning to leave.

In the Mercer report *Living Longer, Better: Understanding Longevity Literacy*, Sonsino identifies other real solutions to help retain 50-and-older employees, including upskilling, building community networks within the company, and making sure that age discrimination is not a part of a company's culture.[38]

Some forward-thinking companies are taking an even more significant step in looking at how longevity is going to impact not just their talent but their whole business. If companies don't adjust their approaches and policies for the 50-and-up workers, not only will they lose current employees, but they will soon lose those who are coming up the ranks.

Ben Legg is the founder of portfolio-collective.com, a UK-based company that focuses on portfolio careers, where people engage in multiple income-earning roles at the same time rather than being beholden to one employer. This idea includes "side hustles," where someone has a main job and one or more smaller gigs in their spare time. But it goes beyond that to include freelancing, contract work, and entrepreneurship.[39] Legg's organization has built a supportive community with more than fourteen thousand members who have access to courses, articles, tools, and events. One of his members landed three different paid work opportunities, as a marketing consultant, a fractional venture partner in a UK security technology company, and a paid mentor.[40] Legg sees this as a major trend in the future of work: "Global forecasts suggest that 50 percent of all professionals will have portfolio careers by 2030."[41]

It's already a trend in the United Kingdom. A study by the UK Department of Education found that 63 percent of adults in England either have a portfolio career or are planning one in the future.[42] While there are no tracking numbers for the United States, Legg's group estimates that it could be as high as 50 percent.

Will the future of the longevity nation become an entirely new kind of work model, with pooled solutions for health insurance and benefits that individuals can buy into? These organizations already exist, including the Freelancers Union and Trupo in the United States, PensionBee in the United Kingdom, Gigacover in the Philippines, and Virtual Freelancer Asia (VFA).

While younger professionals may also decide to have portfolio careers, for people over 50, especially those who have been laid off or downsized, this approach is an ideal way to continue working for an income and for a sense of purpose in their lives.

There's Still More Work to Do

While innovative companies are preparing for the older workforce of the future and Re-Imagineer thought leaders are giving them the insights and tools they need, is the overall business world preparing itself for this massive shift in talent?

It seems that some firms are, but there's still a lot of work to do to get rid of systemic structures that aren't relevant for the twenty-first century. Business leaders need a sense of urgency to get ready for what employees will demand in a longevity nation. Those who are bold in their thinking will reap the benefits of attracting and retaining the best talent for their companies.

there's still a lot of work to do to get rid of systemic structures that aren't relevant for the twenty-first century

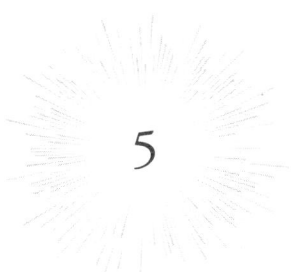

5

How Do You Launch a New Career or Become an Entrepreneur at 50 or Beyond?

In the previous chapter, we briefly discussed reskilling and upskilling as part of company efforts to retain older, experienced workers. But who says that you have to stay within the same company or industry? Or that you need a formal degree from a university to transition to something new?

After a long and successful career in the luxury publishing business, including stints at *The New Yorker* and *Gourmet*, Norman Miller could not have imagined how his life would evolve in his 60s.[1] All he knew was that he was ready to pivot to something new, so he left New York City for the Hudson Valley and got a job at Lowe's in the flooring department. "Soon I was managing plumbing, flooring, paint, and home décor, and there were those in the store that were convinced that I was from the television show *Undercover Boss*," he joked in an email exchange we had in November 2023.[2]

While he enjoyed the work, back surgery prevented him from being able to perform all the lifting required, and he had to rethink his future once more. During his recovery, he saw a job for territory sales at Culligan, the home water systems that deliver cleaner, safer water. He applied and got the job, and after some consolidations and reorganizations, he became the area sales manager with eleven salespeople under his watch. Not only did Miller bring his management skills to his new work, but he is now a proud licensed water specialist and has even talked about water issues on Catskills News Radio. He never imagined he'd become a water expert.[3] In his 60s, Miller found a new path in a field he loves, a complete reinvention that used his acquired skills as he learned a new industry on the job.

There's a high need for critical trade skills in the United States, making this a good possibility for a second or third career in someone's life. Skilled workers such as carpenters, electricians, and plumbers are in much demand: A study by McKinsey & Company found that for many of these roles, annual hiring through 2032 is expected to be more than twenty times the projected increase in net new jobs,[4] meaning there will be a lot of turnover. Although some of this is a byproduct of an aging workforce and fewer younger people who might pursue the trades, imagine if it were turned on its head and people over 50 moved into this as a next act?

While you may not want to become a construction worker, there are lots of low-intensity jobs within the sector that might be perfect for your own reimagination, especially if you have a passion as a weekend craftsperson. Starting something new might include leaning into your accumulated knowledge, like Miller's management skills, or else learning something new that pivots you in a new direction. As life expectancies continue to grow and people realize that a traditional retirement in their mid-60s is an old-fashioned construct, they're thinking about what a post-career life may look like in career 2.0 or as an entrepreneur. And it might be a ten- or twenty-year career. Ask many professionals in their 30s and they will tell you that they expect to have many careers, as they realize they may have much longer lives than their parents and grandparents. A healthy 65-year-old today may live to be 95. That's thirty years that is hard to fill with the proverbial golf games and visits with grandchildren. People need purpose and engagement, not to mention income.

Becoming an Entrepreneur

In the *Wall Street Journal* article "The Investor Betting on People in Their 50s and 60s—Because Older Is Better," journalist Ben Cohen pointed out that older founders have lots of advantages that tend to be overlooked by investors who are obsessed with discovering young talent.

Older entrepreneurs have connections, credibility, experience, and the kind of relationships that can take years to cultivate.[5]

Launching an entrepreneurial business or putting a hobby on supercharge is becoming how many people are building a new chapter in a post-career life. There are lots of resources that you can explore to do the same, including *Start Your Own Business* from the staff of Entrepreneur Media and *Side Hustle: From Idea to Income in 27 Days* by Chris Guillebeau. There are also free courses online, such as those available on Skillshare and Coursera, and your community college may offer in-person training. A simple search may lead you to something that ignites your future.

Older entrepreneurs have connections, credibility, experience, and the kind of relationships that can take years to cultivate

Of those who choose to pursue entrepreneurship, some become consultants or advisors in their existing industries, but there are many others who completely change it up. These Re-Imagineers are hard at work building new identities, personas, and reputations.

Ron Minutella

Ron Minutella went into corporate finance after earning a BA in accounting and an MBA in finance, yet he always had a passion for dance music. In the early 90s, he was introduced to DJ Billy Carroll, who ultimately became his mentor and best friend. He would hang out with him at the DJ booth, absorbing his mixing skills and style. As Minutella gained skills, Carroll got him into the number one DJ record pool in the country.[6] "I would rush from my corporate job to pick up the latest vinyl promo-only and prereleases from all the major record companies," he said. "Billy also helped me secure a Friday night DJ residency at the legendary New York City club, Champs."[7]

Minutella said he was living his best life ever, juggling two careers, his day job during the week and his DJing on the weekend. But ultimately, he had to reevaluate the demands of both jobs and put his DJ role on the back burner to give 150 percent to his finance career. In 2021, he decided it was time to wind down his corporate career to become a full-time professional DJ in his 60s, reclaiming his passion for what excited him.

"Everything had moved to digital, so I had to reimagine my approach, investing a lot of time and energy in researching the latest technology, equipment, and sources for music," he said.[8] He moved to South Florida and used his business skills to think about how he might launch his hobby into a business. He began to secure gigs, filling a niche that was not really being served: a bar/lounge with an NYC underground vibe. He worked within the nonprofit space for efforts like FLoatarama, a group that raises funds to lift up LGBTQ+ youth.

He has become a true Re-Imagineer by transitioning into what gives him the most joy

Today, Minutella has a following of people who only know him as one of the hottest DJs around. He has become a true Re-Imagineer by transitioning into what gives him the most joy, making a living in his new profession. You can hear his music on Soundcloud.com/ronnieminutella.

Yolanda Taylor

Yolanda Taylor spent thirty-one years as a flight attendant for Delta Airlines, but her true passion was fashion. As she became more interested in style and trends, she became the go-to style advisor for friends and family members.[9]

"I understood the struggle that women were going through over 40 as their body shapes changed. I wanted to be the answer and the support that women needed as they navigated their personal style," she said.[10]

In 2018, she started a side hustle called At the Style Table. She began with style blogs and took on some clients as she continued with her day job. By 2021, she decided to invest in the business full-time with virtual styling services, video tips on styling, and more. With the support of her husband, Art, and her family, she stepped out to devote her time to what she envisions as making style accessible to all women, something she says is an essential element of self-care.

Peg Pardini

Peg Pardini is a personal fitness trainer in suburban Pittsburgh, a business that she started in her 30s. Along the way, she took a CPR course, as it was one of the skills she wanted to have should she need it in one of her fitness classes. Once she learned the skill, she decided to take it to the next step and become an instructor, which included in-person training, a test of physical skills, and a written test. In her late 50s, given the physical demands of her profession, Pardini decided to put her years of training to use and reimagine her business. She is moving full-time into CPR and safety instructions for companies and individuals. She works for the American Heart Association and the Red Cross, and she plans to devote her time to teaching this skill to everyone.[11] From one experience taking a CPR class, she now has a thriving business in the space.

Luciano Bernardini de Pace

Often, a business idea can be inspired through the love of something like food, the outdoors, or sustainability. Luciano Bernardini de Pace had a long business career in Milan, but in his 60s, he made a big decision. Since his children were grown and he was newly single, he returned to the origins of his family in Puglia, Italy, where he bought an old palazzo in Bagnolo del Salento and restored it.[12]

The Palazzo Bernardini de Pace is not only his home, but also a luxury destination for travelers to the area. He also decided to start a pasta company. He bought twenty-five hectares of land and chose an ancient wheat, Senatore Cappelli, which has low gluten content. The brand is labeled "Societa Agricola: Luciano Bernardini de Pace, Bagnolo del Salento" and is sold online and in local stores. Food had always been an important part of de Pace's life, and he wanted it to be part of his new life: "My goal is to welcome guests and to cook for them too, not only my pasta but with products from the region. I will also accompany guests to local places in Puglia like Matera or Lecce."[13]

Making a move as bold as his requires a lot of work and, of course, the money to make the leap into your passion project. While you may not be able to self-fund a project, you have a community around you who might be happy to help. If you're truly motivated to turn your hobby into a business, it just takes homework and perseverance to find the money to do it. Who in your family and circle of friends have been your biggest supporters? They may become angel investors or give you a loan. The Small Business Administration (SBA) might be a good route, especially since they have funding for groups such as women-owned businesses, veteran-owned businesses, and more.

you have a community around you who might be happy to help

Wendy Wright

Wendy Wright reimagined herself from working in healthcare to becoming a park ranger in her 50s. It all started when she shifted away from the typical family vacation and chose a solo volunteer week with the Yosemite Conservancy. "This was 100 percent out of my comfort zone! I did strenuous trail work by day and solo camping in the wilderness (with bears) by night. I have never felt more vibrantly alive," she said.[14]

Wright started the process after she was introduced to the "Compass Point" while participating in Camp Reinvention's life-changing twelve-week program for women in midlife and beyond, which was covered in chapter 2. Compass Point is a feeling state. It's your answer to the question, "How do you want to feel about yourself and your life on your very last day?"

It led Wright to a life change in the outdoors, as she wanted to pay attention to moments that evoke a sense of awe and inspiration. Seeing waterfalls and rainbows in her new life's work is only one way that she instills awe into her everyday life.[15]

Adam Weiss

Adam Weiss had a long career as a CEO in the hospitality business but made a major pivot in his 60s. "I led a hospitality organization in lower Manhattan and witnessed 9/11 firsthand. This life-changing event caused my initial shift to leave the corporate world and relocate my wife and children to our upstate home in Woodstock, New York," he explained.[16]

They built a successful bed and breakfast, but his love of vegetable gardening led him to become a certified organic master gardener. "I realized that I had an opportunity to share this skill set with the corporate community, especially as companies were looking to enhance their corporate culture and employee engagement," he said.[17]

Weiss created Pike Lane Gardens, a wellness program that teaches the foundations of organic gardening. Regardless of whether you live in an urban, suburban, or rural setting, he and his team provide seasonal gardening kits, monthly webinars, and garden-to-kitchen classes as part of their teaching techniques.

Now in his mid-60s, Weiss has happily "re-imagined" a new professional direction, and he is sharing his passion with people from around the country. You can see what he is up to at pikelanegardens.com.

Alison Matz

Tapping into that voice in the back of your head that tells you that you want to be your own boss might lead you to become an entrepreneur in the second half of life.

Alison Matz was a media executive who always felt that she was an entrepreneur at heart. Throughout her business career, she was fascinated by what she calls disruptor brands, companies that were taking on category leaders and monopolies with better products and more innovation. In her 50s, she stepped out to launch Skura Style, a lifestyle brand dedicated to kitchen well-being. Their cleaning sponges offer superior performance for consumers, according to Matz.[18]

Matz started the company with her friend Linda Sawyer, whom she had known since second grade. They self-funded the venture when it was in prelaunch to invest in product R&D and prototypes, then raised a seed round cultivated through their professional networks. The investments grew as the business grew over the next ten years. They learned to tap into resources to guide them in areas where they had no expertise. They found experts through informal brain-picking with friends or other like-minded entrepreneurs. Their mission to take on the sponge category had lots of developmental pathways, including a connection with a former IKEA industrial designer, who ultimately became their product and packaging designer. Skura is the Swedish word for "scour" or "scrub."

Launching a business from the ground up is the wildest roller-coaster ride you will ever be on

I asked Matz what it felt like to take the leap into entrepreneurship. She said, "I have often been asked how I had the guts to do this, but now I think it would have been much scarier for me not do it. Launching a business from the ground up is the wildest roller-coaster ride you will ever be on."[19]

Barbara Kotlikoff

Barbara Kotlikoff had a storied career in the beauty and jewelry industry, from Parfums Nina Ricci to Harry Winston (where she was the US managing director) to Monet Jewelry, where she became the global president. When Monet was sold, she decided it was time for a whole new challenge and joined the Paley Center for Media, a nonprofit organization, as the vice president of development, where she spent seven years. From there she moved to New York University to become the assistant dean for development at the Steinhardt School of Culture, Education, and Human Development. She raised more than $60 million in her five-year tenure there, but always had the idea of becoming an entrepreneur, a decision that she finally made at 60.[20]

The Butler's Closet came out of her personal interest in protecting some of her special pieces of clothing, as well as new upholstery, but she couldn't find anything suitable. The company manufactures and sells museum-quality textile conservation items, from garment bags to furniture covers, all made from undyed and unbleached fabrics. "Mine is a business of details—keeping products in stock, introducing new items and marketing to new and repeat customers. It takes a lot of time but is a labor of love," she said.[21]

What Are You Waiting For?

Jumping into the world of entrepreneurship may seem daunting, but as these examples illustrate, it could be one of the best decisions you make. Furthermore, research shows that the number of entrepreneurs over 50 is growing and that they tend to have higher success rates than younger ones. Data from the Kauffman Foundation in 2019 showed that more than 25 percent of new entrepreneurs were between the ages of 55 and 64, a substantial increase from around 15 percent in 1996.[22] According to the Global Entrepreneurship Monitor (GEM), 70 percent of ventures created by people over 50 are still in operation five years after start-up compared to just 28 percent launched by younger entrepreneurs.[23] A study led by Hao Zhao, an associate professor at Rensselaer Polytechnic Institute, found that older entrepreneurs not only experience slightly higher levels of satisfaction but attain greater financial success.[24] The findings are supported by the *Oxford University Press Public Policy and Aging Report* in an article called "Senior Entrepreneurship: The New Normal."[25]

Popular media also provides support for the idea that entrepreneurship shouldn't be limited to the young. According to a *Forbes* article, "Older Entrepreneurs Outperform Younger Founders—Shattering Ageism," the older you get, the higher your chances of success are.[26] It also notes that the most successful founders established expertise in their industry or found success in other jobs before starting their ventures.

But the best way to gain the confidence to take your passion into a business is to look around you. Who do you know who has done it? What can you learn from them that you can apply to your idea? What were the pros and the cons for them? What companies, lenders, and other potential collaborators might help you on your journey?

You'll be surprised at how many people will support and help you when you decide to reimagine your future entrepreneurial path. Ask them to join you for a coffee or a walk or run in the park to share their thoughts. All it takes is the commitment in your own mind to roar forward in a new direction.

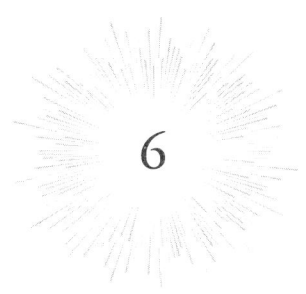

6

Got Money?
Can We Fund a 100-Year Life?

In 1935 in America, life expectancy was 62 years. This was the year Social Security was established as a safety net for older Americans. In those days, there were approximately 7.8 million people who were 65 or older.[1]

Today, there are nearly sixty million Americans aged 65 and over. By 2040, there will be almost eighty million in that age group.[2] With better health and lifestyle choices, living to 90 or 100 is becoming more and more real for many people, not just in the United States but around the world.

Despite this, a study conducted by Voya Financial in early 2025 revealed that just one quarter (24 percent) of Americans believe that they will have saved enough for retirement to live to 100.[3] This percentage is significantly higher among benefits-eligible working Americans at 33 percent, according to Kerry Sette, vice president, head of Consumer Insights and Research at Voya. However, this is still notably short of the 70 percent of Americans who reported wanting to live as long as they possibly can.[4]

The big question—and a legitimate concern—everyone has to ask themselves is "How am I going to fund a 100-year life?" Fortunately, there are a number of Re-Imagineers providing new road maps to answer this question.

The Importance of Financial Literacy

"The majority of Americans don't think their savings will last their lifetime. By a large margin, the number one attribute people are looking for in their retirement plan is ensuring that they won't outlive their savings," said Cyrus Bamji, chief strategy and communications officer at Alliance for Lifetime Income (ALI).[5] The Washington-based organization is a nonprofit 501(c)(6) that educates Americans about the value and importance of having "protected income," such as Social Security, in retirement. Protected income does not include "probable income" such as stock or bond portfolio withdrawals, real estate sales, rental income, or other assets. Ultimately, all forms of liquid and illiquid assets determine an individual's net worth and how they will be able to fund a 90-year or longer life. There are only three forms of protected income that are potentially guaranteed to Americans: Social Security, pensions, and annuities, according to ALI.

> **The majority of Americans don't think their savings will last their lifetime**

ALI has sixteen academics and thought leaders in the retirement space, including such experts as Jason Fichtner, former deputy commissioner of Social Security; personal finance journalist Jean Chatzky, founder and CEO of HerMoney.com; Richard Leider, author and founder of Inventure; and Anne Lester, former portfolio manager and head of retirement solutions for JPMorgan Asset Management's solutions group. These Re-Imagineers are focused on finding new ways to educate consumers and financial planners and on creating policy for a world where financial security is a possibility for everyone, regardless of their socioeconomic level.

At Bank of America Private Bank, president Katy Knox has incorporated new strategies for her sales teams about how to address longevity topics with their clients. "We are at a pivotal moment where lifespan and health span integration is more important than ever. This dynamic is having a meaningful impact on how people are viewing and preparing for later life and in turn, how we are supporting our clients," she said.[6] The strategy includes deeper engagements with multi-generational family members, easier digital tools, and a focus on women. "The industry data shows that 70 percent of women leave the couple's financial planner after the death of her husband. We need to find ways to have more meaningful relationships with them."[7]

According to the Bank of America Institute, an estimated $124 trillion in US wealth is expected to be transferred through 2048. Of the total, $54 trillion will be transferred to surviving spouses, with 95 percent expected to be going to women. Another $74 trillion is expected to go to women in younger generations as wealth is inherited.

"Women generally live longer than men and we need to take more time to get them ready to take on inherited wealth," Knox said. "It doesn't mean investment meetings, but rather incorporating financial knowledge and advice with events in art, sports, or longevity topics."[8]

Russ Hill is the executive chairman of California-based Halbert Hargrove Global Advisors, the chairman of the Stanford Center on Longevity Advisory Council, and the author of *Optimizing Longevity*. His book not only follows the principles of the Stanford Center's New Map of Life, but also offers innovative thinking on how to prepare for financial security for the 100-year life. His methodology, the "Personal Funded Ratio" (PFR), shows you the relationship between what you have in finances, both present and future, and what you expect or have to spend, both present and future. Once you understand what you're working with, you can plan accordingly.[9]

Financial literacy and reimagining how we all think about our finances is having a significant moment in what ALI has termed "the peak 65 zone," a surge of 65-year-olds that will run through 2027.[10] In 2025, an average of 11,400 Americans will turn 65 every day, setting a historic milestone with 4.1 million reaching what has been known as the traditional retirement age.[11] By 2030, the last baby boomer will turn 65, and the cycle will reach those high numbers again in twenty years when the millennial generation moves into that age group. In a study commissioned by ALI's Retirement Income Institute, more than half of the baby boomers turning 65 between 2024 and 2030 have assets of $250,000 or less.[12] And in ALI's 2025 annual *Protected Retirement Income & Planning* study, more than half of Peak 65 consumers (ages 61–65) have investable household assets of less than $100,000.[13]

Many of these people may run out of their savings and be forced to rely on Social Security, which was designed to only replace about 40 percent of a person's annual pre-retirement income, on average, according to Bamji.[14] Add in inflation, healthcare costs, investment performance, and the possibility of living to 90 or 100, and the question "Will my money last?" becomes even more relevant.

"Regardless of your individual socioeconomic status and lifestyle costs, focus on income as the outcome. Whether you're a millionaire or middle income, everyone up and down the socioeconomic scale has the same concerns—will I be able to maintain my lifestyle and will my money last? It's all relative," explained Bamji.[15]

You might be planning on receiving the largest generational transfer of wealth in the history of the world to relieve your financial burden, but not everyone will be so lucky. Still, by 2045, there will be $84–$124 trillion transferred to those fortunate individuals and families who are Generation X, millennials, and younger.[16] A large portion of that will be in North America alone. Approximately $31 trillion will be passed on over the next ten years.[17] "We need to make sure that we are there for the next generation when this happens, getting them ready for what could be a high level of unexpected wealth," said Bank of America's Knox.[18]

That group may have less concern about funding the 100-year life, if they maintain investment strategies to protect their capital and earn decent returns. For others, the concern will be more real. It supports the importance of financial literacy as a lifetime pursuit for everyone. In the United States, the looming issue is the future state of the Social Security system and what kind of reforms might be needed to not only pay out for today's recipients but ensure that it can support future generations as well.

In the United States, the looming issue is the future state of the Social Security system

The Government's Role in Financial Longevity

At the writing of this book, Social Security, Medicare, and other health-related costs make up more than 50 percent of the federal budget, and much of it is core to the financial well-being of millions of

Americans, especially those in lower and middle class groups.[19] Unfortunately, the future of Social Security is in jeopardy, but reforms to extend its viability aren't imminent. When I spoke with Jason Fichtner, he told me that no one in Washington wants to touch the issue of Social Security reform. Since Social Security has no borrowing authority, it will only be able to pay out in benefits from what it collects in payroll taxes and some taxation of the benefits. And if there are no reforms, the reserve will be depleted by 2033, resulting in 20–25 percent cuts in benefits.[20] Fichtner has a few ideas to reimagine the system: "We can't cut our way out of this. There will have to be revenue increases, maybe through payroll taxes, raising the taxable maximum for higher income earners, or other sources of taxes," he said. "Reducing other parts of the federal budget doesn't necessarily free up general funds for Social Security, which is primarily funded by a dedicated payroll tax. Any use of general revenues would have to be legislated, and both sides of the political aisle are concerned that using general revenues to shore up the program might make Social Security more of a welfare program than an earned benefit"[21]

Acknowledging that a 20 percent reduction is not palatable for the American people, Fichtner suggests that other moves might include a reduction of cost-of-living increases or a gradual increase in the full retirement age from 67 to 69 or 70. To accommodate people who cannot work past 62 due to hard labor jobs, he proposes a bump up of minimum benefit for those individuals. Fichtner also likes the idea of allowing Social Security funds to be invested in equities, noting that if that had happened in 1983, the system would be much healthier today. A change in policy to allow a portion to be invested might yield great gains in future years. Right now, the money sits in special-issue Treasury securities, but individuals or banks cannot buy them. Another option might be to reduce benefits for higher income earners.

"What you could do is tax Social Security on the Form 1040 at a different rate. There are different tax rates, like capital gains. Creating a different Social Security tax rate for higher income individuals could be a solution," said Fichtner.[22] According to him, most financial professionals suggest that individuals need a 70–80 percent replacement rate in retirement based on the previous three to five years of working history. Social Security plays an important part in that calculation but is designed to replace only about 40 percent for the average person. Additionally, many Americans are concerned about their financial future overall and how they will have enough income in retirement, both from Social Security and their investments.

In an ALI study, the average age people started receiving Social Security benefits was at 59.2 years old. When asked why they chose to begin receiving benefits before full retirement age, approximately 43 percent of respondents said it was due to a disability or inability to work, 32 percent reported that they needed the income, and 28 percent said that they wanted to take the money early because they were concerned they wouldn't get it otherwise (because it wouldn't be there in the future, benefits would be cut, or they would pass away before reaching full retirement age).[23]

The hard fact is that the earlier someone takes Social Security, the less they will get on a monthly basis for the rest of their life. For example, if someone takes Social Security at 62, it is 30 percent less than what they would get if they waited until age 70. And this is on top of the potential decrease in benefits that looms on the horizon. As a result, it is important not to expect to rely solely on Social Security payments

it is important not to expect to rely solely on Social Security payments

ments. Do everything you can to delay taking them, such as employing a bridge strategy.

Bridging the Gap and Other Long-Term Financial Strategies

Emerson Sprick, associate director of economic policy at the Bipartisan Policy Center, advocates for a Social Security "bridge strategy" to help someone delay taking benefits until they can get their maximum payout.[24] According to Sprick, up to age 70, monthly benefit amounts increase every month they remain unclaimed. In concrete terms, this means that each year of delay nets a real return of 7–8 percent. A bridge strategy uses personal and retirement savings to help someone bridge the gap from 62 until they might claim Social Security at a later age. During that time, they may work part-time or become an entrepreneur as their benefits build.

Fichtner adds that a five-year annuity is also a way to bridge to age 70.[25] Another idea is to buy a deferred annuity that kicks in at 85, when you might need additional income.

In 2024, Prudential Financial, in collaboration with Fidelity Investments, launched Prudential SimplyIncome, a new single-premium immediate annuity within employer-based retirement plans.[26] It's a great example of companies thinking in Re-Imagineer terms by offering an innovative idea that provides a new decumulation option for participants who want a predictable retirement income solution.

In his book, Russ Hill recommends other financial moves that can help with long-term security. "Longevity pooling" is an approach that combines the assets of a group of people who are the same age, so the survivors see their distributions increase over time as the number of participants decreases.[27] They include deferred payout annuities or single premium annuities. The Qualified Longevity Annuity Contract (QLAC) is now part of many retirement programs in the deferred classification, while in the single annuity, investors contribute to what becomes a guaranteed income for life.

Another approach is the "tontine," which Hill describes as a shared annuity where investors pool money and receive payouts from the pool. An individual receives payments until their death, when the remaining amount goes to the remaining participants. Tontines are managed by a fiduciary organization, such as Tontine Trust Advisors or Colorado-based Savvly.

Ultimately, however, which financial longevity policies are in place and which financial products are available depends on Washington. Those policymakers who will lead the charge on change are the true Re-Imagineers. Richard Neal (D-MA) and Edward Markey (D-MA) are two members of Congress who have advocated for retirement security and reforms, including supporting the SECURE 2.0 Act of 2022. It aims to increase retirement savings and participation through a series of provisions that include catch-up contributions and requiring employers to automatically enroll new employees into 401(k) programs.[28]

In a letter to his investors, BlackRock CEO Larry Fink lamented that nearly half of American workers have no pensions and zero in a 401(k) plan, ringing the alarm on the importance of this topic.[29] The good news is that many companies have already adopted automatic enrollment on a voluntary basis. A growing number of states from Illinois to Washington to Colorado have begun mandating that workers have access to a retirement savings vehicle, but as of July 2025, only twenty states have mandated retirement programs.[30]

Another important policy area concerns how older adults cover health-related costs, including long-term care. In September 2024, I spoke with Gopi Shah Goda about this issue. Goda has a PhD in economics from Stanford University, has worked at the Stanford Institute for Economic Policy Research and the National Bureau of Economic Research, and in 2025 joined the Brookings Institution as a senior fellow and became the director of their Retirement Security Project.[31] She has spent a large part of her career researching the economics of aging and how people make decisions about saving for retirement and healthcare as they age: "One of the biggest challenges is that people are very unprepared for financing long-term care. There is not a policy solution at the moment. Care is oftentimes Medicaid, and someone needs to meet stringent income and asset thresholds. People sometimes get there by essentially impoverishing themselves by paying for long-term care."[32]

In her year with the Council of Economic Advisers at the White House, Goda saw how research can influence policy. She is interested in the intersection of evidence-based research and policy making to help improve financial well-being for older adults. In our conversation, she explained that she is thinking about how people can use the tax code to finance some of their healthcare spending: "An individual can deduct medical and dental expenses that exceed 7.5 percent of their adjusted gross income. Not everyone who is eligible actually takes advantage of it. How can we figure out the barriers and frictions that are there, especially for needier taxpayers? One question is how much

people are very unprepared for financing long-term care

of this is being used as a mechanism to finance long-term care and who is making use of that provision to do so?" [33]

In her reimagined thinking, Goda is hoping to study how the tax code and medical deductions may reduce financial burden as people age, noting that there needs to be a lot more research on the subject.

Financial Resilience Around the World

Ensuring one has sufficient funds for their later years is not just an American issue; it's also an important global one, as developed countries continue to see life expectancies grow. In several Asian countries, life expectancy for women is already hovering around 90.[34]

Haleh Nazeri of the World Economic Forum coauthored a report with Rich Nuzum, executive director of Investment and global chief investment strategist at Mercer. The report, "Longevity Economy Principles: The Foundation for a Financially Resilient Future," identifies six principles to address the challenges of aging populations and promote financial resilience for everyone:

- **Principle 1:** ensuring financial resilience across key life events
- **Principle 2:** providing universal access to impartial financial education
- **Principle 3:** prioritizing healthy aging as foundational for the longevity economy
- **Principle 4:** evolving jobs and lifelong skill building for a multigenerational workplace
- **Principle 5:** designing systems and environments for social connection and purpose
- **Principle 6:** intentionally addressing longevity inequalities, including across gender, race, and class[35]

"Our goal is to ensure that people don't retire into poverty, and what does that look like," said Nazeri, adding that preventative healthcare is critical. "We don't want people to save all this money and then have to spend it all on healthcare."[36]

In the report, the authors showcase some best practices around the world that are helping build toward a reimagined future for financial well-being. For example, in Denmark, financial education has been a core part of student curriculum since 2015. Each year, around twenty thousand students participate in Danish Money Week, focusing on financial education. The country has one of the highest financial literacy rates in the world, at 71 percent.[37]

According to Nazeri, employers are where most people are going for financial education and to understand how to stay solvent for a long life. She cited companies like Manulife in Canada and Mercer and AXA in France as companies that are doing it right.[38] "The private sector in general is way ahead of the game. Governments are the ones that are kind of in waiting mode," she said.[39] Other great programs to address the issue include MoneySense in Singapore, which helps Singaporeans manage their money and make sound financial decisions; the John Hancock Vitality program, which rewards people for everyday healthy activities; and a program designed by Swiss Re called Flex58+, where an employee can flexibly reduce working time before retirement while their previous base salary is still insured in the pension fund. Then they can move into an advisory role post-retirement on a contract basis.[40]

Based on a 2023 S&P survey of eighty-one countries, governments that fail to change aging-related fiscal policies will run a deficit of 9.1 percent of GDP by 2060, up from 2.4 percent in 2025. The World Economic Forum predicts that people might outlive their retirement savings by eight to twenty years, with women as the most at-risk group.[41]

According to data from studies like the S&P Global FinLit Survey, the top countries for financial literacy include Norway, Sweden, Denmark, Canada, and the Netherlands, all of which are committed to teaching financial skills to both students and adults.[42] One of the goals of the S&P study is to inform policymakers, regulators, and the private sector on how to develop effective financial education policies and programs. With populations living longer than ever, it is a critical time to create financial literacy in every country around the world. A part of that will include a new breed of financial adviser, who will view the 100-year life as the target age for making an individual's money last but who will also expand the conversation to make sure their clients lead a purposeful life with that financial security.

A Holistic Approach

One such financial adviser is Mark T. Johnsen, founder of Wealth Architects in Mountain View, California. Johnsen has spent more than thirty years working with more than four hundred individuals and families to help them achieve a combination of financial security and lifetime fulfillment.[43] As the "chief wealth architect," his philosophy is that wealth also means well-being, which means fulfillment and meaning in one's life: "Our architectural metaphor is to help our clients with building blocks which include finances, but also health, mind, body, and spirit. Our job is to help our clients align their money with their values."[44]

For example, if a client has an interest in sustainability, Johnsen will ask how they are putting that interest into practice in their daily lives. If they answer that they have installed a solar panel system for their home, Johnsen might suggest investing in companies or funds with a commitment to ESG values.

Another example is how someone may want to translate their interest in philanthropy into an overall approach that considers more than money. If they don't have the funds to donate, they can express their values by giving their time and expertise to something that matters to them.

Johnsen's holistic approach is called Design for a Wealthier Life, and the human elements are as important to him as the financial ones. "If someone is just focused on maximizing their money, I don't want to work with them. Our company of twenty-five individuals share the same belief," he said.[45]

Like Johnsen, Craig Lyman is part of this growing breed of financial advisers who don't want to just focus on the money. He and his wife run a financial advisory firm based in Las Vegas, and they now integrate lifestyle discussions with their clients that include how they want to spend the second half of their lives, especially if they live to 100.[46] "We are focused on that because many of our clients retire, and they end up in bad places. We are now focused on helping them have a meaningful transition into a fulfilling life in combination with what they have saved and invested," Lyman explained.[47]

Nearly 60 percent of Lyman's national client base is 50–69 years old, which he believes is the right time to bring these conversations to the forefront. "With many of our clients, this approach is changing how they think about their future lives. It's holistic planning that is helping them make both financial and lifestyle decisions," he said.[48]

Lyman was a part of the first cohort in Columbia University's Wealth Management master's program, which was launched in 2001. He is currently on the faculty in the program as a lecturer and is bringing his holistic planning into his curriculum. Not only is he a Re-Imagineer in how he approaches financial advising but he is now proselytizing a new approach for those moving into the field. That's the big idea for the future: combining financial literacy and security with a well-thought-out lifespan that puts your assets to work with your life goals. As money and wealth managers, Johnsen and Lyman are helping build the components of the new longevity nation.

That's the big idea for the future: combining financial literacy and security with a well-thought-out lifespan that puts your assets to work with your life goals

Financial Planning for All

While we focus on our health span for a better lifespan, our wealth span is equally important. For this reason, everyone should have a financial adviser regardless of their income and assets. It can be a local banker, a knowledgeable family member or friend, or someone at their company who can help guide them to a secure financial future. But it should be done in concert with a deep discussion about how they want to live the second half of their lives and their ability to afford it. It may mean they will have to work longer or part-time or reduce illiquid assets into usable funds. Some people may need to rethink what they are able to do. Ultimately, the plan has to be a combination of knowing one's financial numbers and asking if they are aligned to live the 90- or 100-year life. It's up to the individual to take this on for their pathway to meaningful longevity. Teaching that to our children now will help them over a longer life.

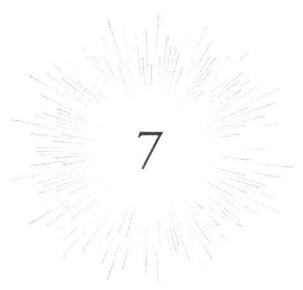

7

Creativity: It Should Never Stop

Paul Theroux is one of my favorite American writers. You might know some of his most famous works: *The Mosquito Coast* or *The Great Railway Bazaar* or *Dark Star Safari*. He has also written short stories, magazine articles, essays, and so much more. One that you'll want to read is his *New Yorker* essay "Facing Ka'ena Point," which contains his reflections on turning 80.

Now in his mid-80s, he continues to be as prolific as ever. When I reached out to him to tell him I was working on a book about longevity and how creativity can continue to thrive as one ages, he reminded me that Picasso never stopped creating, and neither did da Vinci. Somerset Maugham was active into his 80s, ditto Doris Lessing. Ned Rorem was composing music in his 90s, and Philip Glass continues to be active in his 80s.[1]

I was curious how he felt about his creativity now. When I asked him if it was different than when he was in his 60s and 70s, he responded, "I have always felt that the key to creativity is continuity—working uninterruptedly in as much serenity as is available—because the imagination expands with concentration. In other words, don't stop. I have not stopped, and my age has not mattered."[2]

When I asked him where he finds his inspiration for a new project, he said, "The germ of inspiration arises from one's inner life, one's past—and in an older creative person the past is greater, with so much more to stimulate thought. The greatest gift for a creative writer is the ability to listen (and remember) and to observe closely (and remember)—these require patience and humility and reflection, which are almost absent in the young, fairly rare generally, but often traits of older people."[3]

Theroux recommended that I read Sir Kenneth Clark's essay "The Artist Grows Old," Simone de Beauvoir's book *The Coming of Age*, and a book by Nicholas Delbanco called *Lastingness: The Art of Old Age*. All of them deal with the subject of old age and creativity.

Another one of my favorite writers is 82-year-old Isabel Allende, who produces a new work almost every year, including her 2025 novel *My Name is Emilia del Valle*. Her TED Talk "How to Live Passionately—No Matter Your Age" has had more than 4 million views. One of her great comments is that "the spirit never ages."[4] As a creative writer, she continues with her craft, delighting readers like me and millions of others with her beautiful storytelling.

Theroux and Allende are just two examples of creatives who continue to express themselves well into their later years. They are joined by other role models, including Gerhard Richter, a painter in his 90s who continues to work in his native Germany.[5] Helen Mirren and Harrison Ford have thriving careers in their 80s. Eileen Kramer was an Australian dancer and choreographer who died in 2024 at the age of 100 and was known as one of the oldest working dancers.[6]

I asked Theroux if he thought people could begin a creative journey after the age of 50. "You can 'begin' the creative journey, but it won't be easy, because the apprenticeship takes so long. Nonetheless, that should not be a deterrent. My advice would be to get busy, read, write, paint, sculpt—it will matter more than playing golf," he answered.[7]

get busy, read, write, paint, sculpt—it will matter more than playing golf

It's good advice when you consider that Frank McCourt published his first book, *Angela's Ashes*, at the age of 66 and won the Pulitzer Prize.[8] Similarly, Delia Owens was 69 when she finished her first novel, *Where the Crawdads Sing*, a book that stayed on the *New York Times* bestseller list for 168 weeks, sold fifteen million copies, and became a successful movie.[9] Grandma Moses began painting at 78 and lived to 101. At 83, her painting *Sugaring Off* sold at Christie's auction house for $1,360,000.[10]

In his book *The Real Work: On the Mystery of Mastery*, Adam Gopnik dispels the myth that we can't learn new things as we age. His thesis is that we can accomplish anything at any age if we set our minds to it through a series of learning scenarios. Over the course of the book, Gopnik tells the reader how he takes on new creative pursuits like ballroom dancing, drawing, and even boxing lessons.[11]

The takeaway? If you were told that you couldn't learn to play the piano over 50, think again. In so many ways, we block our own potential creative expressions through our own self-imposed ageism.

The Benefits of Creativity

Aside from actually learning to play the piano over 50, there are other benefits to taking on a creative endeavor, including improved brain health, better stress management, and a feeling of accomplishment. Putting our neuroplasticity to work to learn more complex tasks keeps our brains active and engaged according to a report on SmartWellness called "How Creativity Echoes in Health." Creative activities engage multiple parts of your brain, building connections between them. Your prefrontal cortex kicks in when you're planning your approach and solving problems. Your default mode network is active when you're daydreaming. And your limbic system governs the emotional response you have to your creative ideas and output. The report also referenced a study in *Neurology* that found that people who engaged in artistic or creative activities in middle or later life were 73 percent less likely to develop mild cognitive impairment than those who did not.[12] In addition, a fourteen-year study called the English Longitudinal Study of Ageing at the University College London found that adults who frequently engaged in "receptive arts" (such going to plays or museums) had a 31 percent lower risk of dying than those who did not.[13]

LifeConnect24, a company based in Britain, suggests older people learn how to play either the piano, guitar, ukulele, harmonica, or drums.[14] But I would add, pick any instrument and open up your inner musical talent.

we all have some type of creative gene in us that we should explore or develop

I've always believed that we all have some type of creative gene in us that we should explore or develop. An October 1976 *Time* magazine article quoted Picasso as saying, "Every child is an artist. The problem is how to remain an artist once he grows up."[15] Although there is no primary source for this quote, I sure do like the sentiment. Fortunately, many organizations can help you begin walking your creative pathway. Some of them are in person, others are online, and some offer both options. Regardless, there is undoubtedly an organization out there that is perfect for you. It could even be one of these.

The Julliard School

When I went to The Juilliard School campus in New York City to meet with John-Morgan Bush, the dean of Juilliard Extension, it was apparent that he is a Re-Imagineer who is on a mission to promote creative aging and make sure we keep that childhood sensibility alive. The world-famous Juilliard School, a private performing arts conservatory, has three key areas it focuses on: Preparatory for young artists 6–18 years old, a college that offers undergraduate and graduate degrees, and the Extension program, which has approximately 1,300 students—50 percent of whom are over 65 years old.[16] While many of their courses are topics like "The Compositional Through Lines from Beethoven to Bill Monroe" or other historical perspectives, Bush has been focused on building out the participatory program that now includes adult classes in ballet, drama, voice, and more. "We want to help people pick up on a passion that they had in their younger years or else discover something for the first time. The goal is to help adults ignite their curiosity about the arts and express them in their individual way," he said.[17]

A good example is the Beginner's Piano program, which according to Bush can be for someone who has never put their finger on a keyboard before. The school has three classes, with ten to twelve people in each one. When I asked him if the students who attend their programs or earn certificates in core musical skills, music composition, or music production are doing it for their own interest or have ambitions to move into a creative field as their next chapter, he said both. "One of our students studied composition and orchestration and would love to have his works read, performed, or recorded. Another one had a play produced in New Orleans, but some do it for the joy of it. We want to provide the pathway to creativity for anyone's intention."[18]

He also believes that arts organizations play a role in the longevity sector, particularly as we live longer: "Most of the focus is on post-acute care or therapy. We believe that music and the arts can be used as a preventative, non-clinical intervention, especially for people who are combating loneliness or isolation."[19]

He's been working with Jill Sonke, PhD, director of research initiatives in the Center of the Arts in Medicine at the University of Florida, to produce research that confirms the role of the arts in promoting healthier aging.

Juilliard Extension is one of the few arts organizations with a focus on creative aging. As more and more people move into their 60s, 70s, and beyond, Bush is reimagining what it might mean for individuals and society at large.

The Wallis Annenberg GenSpace

When you step inside the sleek and modern Audrey Irmas Pavilion in the Koreatown section of Los Angeles, the last thing you would expect to find is a so-called "senior center." This is the next generation of the concept, though. The Wallis Annenberg GenSpace is a Re-Imagineer space that appeals to all ages. The philanthropist Wallis Annenberg created it to promote the idea of intergenerational engagement, encourage creativity, and blow up the stereotypes around aging. The innovative, airy space encourages all types of activities—not the typical programming you might find in other centers. "We have more than eighty-five classes a week from fitness to technology training, horticultural work, art classes, and more," explained Christopher Leech, the GenSpace's director.[20]

Leech and his team have designed a slate of programming that requires their members to come on a regular basis. It helps build community and reduces isolation. "We have mothers and daughters who take classes together in art, dance, and more," he said.[21]

The GenSpace is a future-looking way to encourage creativity while also fostering new ways to learn.

The Tent Theater Company

The Tent Theater Company was founded by Tim Sanford—who spent twenty-five years at Playwrights Horizons—and his wife, Aimée Hayes, the former producing artistic director of Southern Rep Theater in New Orleans. Together, these Re-Imagineers nurture, support, and advocate for older American playwrights age 60 and up.[22] The *New York Times* article "The Next Hot Playwright? They Prefer the Ones Who Cooled Off" states, "To [Sanford], though, age is an overlooked element of diversity—one that comes with accumulated knowledge of the human experience, and for which there is, and must be, room."[23]

Stagebridge

Stagebridge is an Oakland, California–based nonprofit that also focuses on including older adults in the performing arts. Their Performing Arts Institute offers courses in theater, acting, dancing, music, and more. They have produced more than thirty-five original works, as well as hundreds of workshops and performances by their students. They welcome students equally whether they participate for the sheer joy of it or hope to become a late-in-life movie star. The positivity of Stagebridge's mission to celebrate and enrich lifelong learners shows us what is possible for a creative future.[24]

Talent Is Timeless

If you are a New Yorker, you can participate in the "Talent Is Timeless" competition, a program created by the New York City Department for the Aging. According to Michael Ognibene, the first deputy commissioner and chief operating officer of the organization, the competition is a series of local, regional, and boroughwide shows that include singing, dancing, poetry, comedy, and more.[25] More than a thousand people participate, and there is a citywide finale showcasing the top three acts from each borough. In 2024, the winner was 61-year-old Rosemarie Hameed, who dazzled the audience with her singing voice. "I came to life after the age of 60," she said after accepting her well-earned trophy.[26]

Ognibene and his team also oversee Intergenerational Groove, which is a dance party held in New York's Foley Square for more than a thousand participants of all ages. GROOVE NYC, which leads the dancing, is a nonprofit organization that uses creativity, music, movement, dance, and art for social change, particularly within generations. In 2025, the GROOVE added Laughter Yoga, which involves a series of movement and breathing exercises to promote deliberate laughter. According to Ognibene, the session (led by Patrick Welage, a retired professor of theology, philosophy, and theatre arts who is now a certified Laughter Yoga teacher) reduces stress, makes the immune system stronger, and creates positive mindfulness.[27]

Online Learning Opportunities to Boost Creativity

Regardless of where you live, you can tap into the flourishing online programs available to anyone. You can do it in your own home, often at your own pace. It is more affordable than many in-person programs (not to mention saving on commuting costs), yet still creates a learning environment. Whether you want to learn how to write a novel, paint a picture, play an instrument, compose a song, or photograph the world, there are numerous opportunities for online learning. In some instances, you might even have the chance to learn from famous professionals. Here are just a few examples of online platforms that offer programs that can aid you in your creative pursuits:

- MasterClass
- Udemy
- Novelry
- Coursera
- New Masters Academy
- YouTube

- International Center of Photography
- School of Photography, UK
- School of Photography, Singapore
- Muench Workshops
- Santa Fe Workshops

Regardless of whether you pursue learning through one of these platforms or somewhere else, the benefits of creative pursuits can't be overstated. All it takes is a search for your area of interest, and you'll find offerings from around the world or in your own community.

Creative Re-Imagineers Worth Meeting

I'm always on the hunt for Re-Imagineers who either reignited a creative passion or took on a new one at midlife and found fulfillment and happiness doing it. I love to find Re-Imagineers who are breaking through barriers and expanding the creative world in ways that make it possible for everyone to create until the end of their lives. Oftentimes it is people who have reclaimed an interest from their younger lives, like writing, but many times it is a new pursuit, like sculpting.

the world is filled with incredibly inspiring stories of people who move into creative passions in the second halves of their lives

Fortunately, the world is filled with incredibly inspiring stories of people who move into creative passions in the second halves of their lives. Some dream of having their own art show, selling their screenplay to Netflix, or writing their first novel. Others do it simply for their own enjoyment and fulfillment. Here are a few of the Re-Imagineers who have participated in creative endeavors in unique and powerful ways.

Alex Rotas, Photographer
Alex Rotas lives in Bristol, England, and is an ambassador for Active Ageing Bristol, which promotes increased physical activity

for people over 50. An academic by background, when she turned 60 she had an epiphany when she couldn't find images of older athletes. It led to her buying a camera, hiring a photography tutor, and learning about masters sports programs.[28]

"I traveled to championships where competitors and teams compete in five-year age bands from 35+ right up to 105+," she said.[29]

She started photographing these athletes, which led to sharing the images with friends and small groups, which then led to talks at schools and corporations. That then led to exhibitions and social media.

"I've photographed thousands of individuals over fifteen years who are masters athletes in swimming, cycling, basketball, hockey, rowers, and more. I've also photographed skydivers who range from POPS (Parachutists Over Phorty) to JONS (Jumpers Over Ninety)," she said.[30]

Rotas made a film following four female British masters athletes aged 69–84 with filmmaker Danielle Sellwood of Find It Film. "We called the film *Younger* to reflect the fact that, every five years, when an athlete enters a new age category, they become the youngster in the group, whether they are 35 or 40, 85 or 90," she explained.[31]

Rotas never expected her original foray into photography to lead her to an entirely new creative profession and passion, but that's what can happen when you take a first step. Her work can be seen at alexrotasphotography.co.uk.

Hers is only one story of creativity.

Alissa Randall, Photographer

Alissa Randall is another Re-Imagineer who pursued creativity later in life. For years, Randall had a successful career as a chief marketing officer for a number of organizations, but then her position was eliminated, which she said "turned out to be a wonderful gift."[32]

That same afternoon, she started her headshot photography business, something that she had been considering for a while:

> When I was thinking about starting the business, I chatted with a coach, Marissa Fernandez. I told her I wanted to be that 70-year-old looking back on an incredible career. She asked me what words I would use to describe the older me. I said: moxie, creative, energetic, sophisticated, smart with business, empathetic, strong, and inspiring. She simply said, you're all those words now. I took that and ran with it.[33]

While she had always loved photography in her downtime, she knew nothing about headshot photography. A call to her local photography equipment store connected her to the rep, Cliff Hauser, for some lighting equipment that she had bought. She asked him if he would teach her how to use the equipment, which he did. She launched "All About Headshots" in 2022 and is thriving in her new creative profession.

Jonathan Fisher, Photographer/Videographer

Jonathan Fisher worked in the transportation business for his whole career. Among many other things, he designed an easily updatable bus stop information module, including both a map showing connections to other routes and algorithm-based arrival times—an early application of computer tech in the public-facing transit system. Guide-a-Ride would go on to become the industry standard.[34]

At 50, he decided to retire from that profession, but he was far from done. He always believed that one of his innate creative skills was being a good storyteller. He went on to work at the ad giant Ogilvy and then the NYC Housing Authority, when he learned that a former colleague and fellow Re-Imagineer, George Carrano, had started a nonprofit dedicated to participatory photography called Seeing for Ourselves. "Taking advantage of my administrative role in public housing, I pitched the agency executive the idea of the nonprofit delivering programming in the projects," Fisher said during our interview. "Positive imagery created by those with lived experience would counter the generation-long focus of crime and disrepair."[35]

Then Chelsea Davis, who had conducted a participatory program in the cancer ward of St. Louis Children's Hospital, amassed a collection of photographs that might change the narrative around public housing. At 63 and with "retirement from work never in the cards,"[36] Fisher, along with Davis and Carrano, decided to produce a book on the project. The result, which they titled *Project Lives*, was incredibly well-received and amassed a number of awards. The late President Jimmy Carter even gave his support. The book also led to more funding from the city and the state.

The trio decided to take the practice to the probation agency, as its clients had also been laboring under scornful media coverage for a generation, according to Fisher. Video interviews led to the idea to create a film project, and Fisher began viewing Ken Burns films for inspiration. The resulting film about New York City probation is called *In a Whole New Way*. It has been welcomed into more than two hundred venues globally and was screened by PBS. It amassed more than eighty awards. A companion book was published shortly thereafter.

Start with what you know

"My advice is to—well, just do it. What do you have to lose? Start with what you know, like storytelling in my case. Then see if you can expand it from there," Fisher said.[37]

John Kneapler, Painter

The Art Students League of New York has been in existence for 150 years, and according to John Kneapler, a painter and member of the board, almost every famous artist in New York has gone there on their way to becoming famous, including Jasper Johns, Jackson Pollock, Maxfield Parrish, and Norman Rockwell.[38]

"It's a wonderful place because you are painting alongside people from 8 to 100 years old, from all walks of life and economic backgrounds. You pay for a class by the month and it's affordable," explained Kneapler.[39]

The league's classes include painting, watercolors, portraiture, sculpture, welding, and more. And while most of it is in person, there are online courses too.

Kneapler's own story fits the profile of the adult Re-Imagineer, returning to something that he loved as a child—painting. His parents dissuaded him from pursuing a career as a painter, so he embarked on a different kind of creative profession in the graphic design world. When he was in his late 40s, he decided to return to painting while running his successful, award-winning company. "I started painting in my apartment, but then I decided to go to the Art Students League on Tuesday nights. Then I went on Tuesdays and Saturdays and pretty soon added Sunday," he said. "I do large abstract landscapes made out of acrylics and when I go on vacation, I take my watercolors." [40]

While Kneapler has traditional art shows, he also sells his work on Instagram. One of his watercolors sold fifty copies within two weeks. When I asked him if he was making a living as a painter he said, "When I was working, I took a month off to paint and started worrying about money. I've disassociated that I don't care if I make money or not. It's the joy of making the art."[41]

Tina Woods, DJ

If you really love to dance, you might be inspired by Re-Imagineer Tina Woods. At 60, she became a techno DJ and has her own club nights called Longevity Rave.[42] Her day job is in health technology and innovation in the field of longevity. She is the founder and CEO of Business for Health, bringing health into ESG mandates to support long-term sustainable innovation and investment in preventative health and care. As a longevity Re-Imagineer, she has been director of the All Party Parliamentary Group for Longevity in the United Kingdom and is the healthy longevity champion for the National Innovation Centre for Ageing there. She also wrote a book called *Live Longer with AI: How Artificial Intelligence Is Helping Us Extend Our Healthspan and Live Better Too.*

Married with three grown sons, she and her husband have grown even closer thanks to her love of dancing and music, as he now joins her in her clubbing efforts. Today, Woods organizes longevity raves around the world, using her love of music as a way to connect with people of all generations. That's her side hustle, as she continues her important longevity work at Business for Health.

Don Loftus, Playwright

Don Loftus had a successful career as the president of several major beauty companies.[43] He was the chairman of the Fragrance Foundation and revered as an industry leader. However, he had a burning creative passion that had been in him since he took his first trip to New York in high school. "A teacher took us on a trip, when I saw four Broadway shows, and I was hooked. I started writing plays in high school with my friend, Mark O'Donnell, who would eventually go on to write the book for the musical *Hairspray*," he said.[44]

While Loftus went on to a business career, he would wake up at 4 AM and write until 7 AM before going to work as a beauty executive. After work and on the weekends, he and his wife would go to the theater to see nearly every production.

When he decided it was time to step out of his career to "rewire" at the age of 64, the decision as to what he would do next was pretty evident. His goal was to unleash his creativity as a playwright, and he has gone at it with full force.

His work has been presented on stages across America, the United Kingdom, India, Australia, and Sweden, as well as in more than a hundred play festivals. He even won the W. Keith Hedrick National Playwriting Award. He joined the board of the Dramatist Guild Foundation and works with other writers, as he continues to write plays at 70. In 2024, his full-length psychodrama, *PER*, was produced by the LAB Theater Project in Tampa, Florida, and in 2025, his work appeared in more than a dozen places from Monterey, California, to New York City. Loftus plans to spend the rest of his life recapturing his boyhood passion for the theater as his full-time work.

Creativity Until the End

Creativity in any form is something that we can all do until the ends of our lives. All of us can begin creating anytime as a hobby or decide to make it a full-time pursuit, like Loftus. Maybe you have already developed a great creative expression like singing or dancing and now you are looking for an outlet to express it.

engaging with creativity on any level is as meaningful to a healthy lifespan as exercise, diet, and community are

If you don't have a creative outlet at the moment, I hope that you are curious about doing something creative or at least experiencing something creative. As previously mentioned, engaging with creativity on any level is as meaningful to a healthy lifespan as exercise, diet, and community are. If you are not doing anything creative at the moment, put that into your longevity lifestyle curriculum. Pick your lane and go full speed ahead. And remember, creativity is something that you can pursue until your last day on earth.

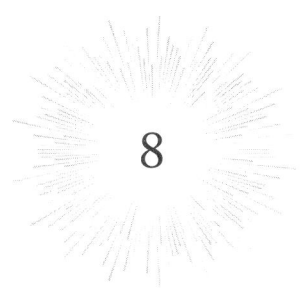

8

Advertising and Media in the Age of the New Longevity

For forty years I had a front row seat in the New York media world, working on the business side of three major publishing companies: Fairchild, Condé Nast, and Hearst. At 34, I became the youngest publisher in the industry at *GQ*, then climbed the ranks to senior and executive vice president roles, before spending ten years as the president and publishing director of Hearst Magazines.

Since advertising revenue was the main source of money for our business, my role was interacting with marketers, advertising agencies, media buyers, and more. I met with CEOs, CMOs, advertising directors, creative directors, trade and consumer press, public relations and publicity people, and anyone else who made up the media ecosystem. I also spent several years as the chairman of the Magazine Publishers of America, which took me to Capitol Hill and other places. All those experiences could be rolled up into their own book, as I got to see it all: the good, the bad, and the ugly.

It was a heady time in the magazine business, before Google, Meta, and Amazon got into the game and the digital disruption took over. But the magazine world and every other media format evolved, survived, and continue to attract audiences that value their brands and trustworthy storytelling.

The marketing and advertising world evolved, too, adapting to new ways to communicate on all kinds of digital platforms. We also had new ways to measure the return on investment of advertising spend.

But during this process, many companies missed a massive megatrend that was right in front of them, leaving tens of millions of dollars on the table. The majority of the advertising world has been way behind in recognizing and acting on how consumers over 50 have changed in radical ways as both buyers of products and users of media. For an industry that prides itself on always being *au courant*, it's an enigma. Actually, it is age-phobia, and it thrives in the advertising world. As Erica Kwok, senior VP and general manager at Estée Lauder said, "In the US, there is a glorification of youth that missed other global perspectives, particularly in Asia, where there is more of a glorification of the wisdom and experience of age."[1]

The media and advertising world has had an obsession with youth which some call the 18-to-34-year-old syndrome, meaning marketers prioritize them for their products. The belief was that you had to get younger people into your brand consideration. It would then turn them into your loyal consumers for the rest of their lives. The idea worked until it didn't.

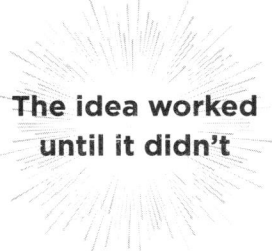

The idea worked until it didn't

John Dick, founder and CEO of CivicScience, the best-in-class next-generation survey and data company, said it best: "The spending capacity of the 50-plus group is something of a no-brainer. They constantly try new things. In fact, over the last decade, there has been a 34 percent increase in trying new brands in this group. They are also market mavens. They try new things, oftentimes learning about them on the internet or social media, and they tell all of their friends about it."[2]

In the ROAR forward survey mentioned in an earlier chapter, 87.7 percent of consumers age 50 and up disagreed with the statement that their brand choices were in place once they hit their mid-50s.[3] In fact, 97.5 percent said that they had bought a new brand within the prior six months. More than 60 percent said they discovered new brands from social media, and more than 60 percent said they avoid brands that have old-fashioned images of people over 50 in their advertising.

So, why do marketers continue to ignore the 50-and-older market, especially since it represents nearly $9 trillion in spending power and would be the third-largest country in the world in GDP? [4] Most people would say that this obsession started when the baby boomers were in their teens and twenties. After all, they were the mega generation of youth at the time, the "Me Generation" that spent a lot of money on themselves. Marketers loved them, and they became the target for all kinds of goods and services. The generation helped build brands like Nike, Reebok, MTV, and *Rolling Stone*. They were a money machine that paid off.

But that concept, which started in the 1970s, led to fifty years of ingrained thinking in marketing, advertising, and creative circles. The chase focused on the cool factor of what younger groups were interested in, and that meant that only younger people knew the answers. In the advertising creative world, you were already viewed as a dinosaur in your 40s, put out to pasture as not being "current." In many sectors like luxury retail and fashion, the photographers, stylists, and designers have become so insular to themselves that they only focus on models and influencers under 30 to represent brands. Often, it is a reflection of their own self-defined cool factor. The problem is that the customers of many of these brands, those who have the money to spend, are well over 40 and really don't relate to images of 25-year-olds.

According to David Sable, the vice-chairman of Stagwell, a global marketing and communications group, "The problem is that people in agencies believe that to be modern and smart, there has to be a focus on younger people. Ten years ago, it was all about the millennials and now the obsession is with Gen Z and Alpha."[5]

The antiquated thinking has been that accomplished and stylish 50-year-old women want to be inspired by these young models, when in fact they see amazing, stylish women over 50 as their role models.

Ruth La Ferla is a former full-time reporter for the *New York Times* who still contributes on fashion, cultural, and societal trends. According to her, "In fashion, true age inclusivity is rare. A high-end campaign may well zero in on an iconic figure—Maggie Smith or Charlotte Rampling, or for that matter, a super-stylized Debbie Harry, who recently vamped for a Gucci campaign. Showcasing celebrities in their 70s or 80s seems a stunt primarily conceived to generate buzz."[6] La Ferla suggested that marketers and traditional media should consider following the lead of TikTok and Instagram figures like Grece Ghanem, a 60-year-old microbiologist turned influencer who demonstrates that style is not limited to the young. "Alternatively, they might mingle older models casually and indiscriminately with others of varying ages in imagery that sends a more authentic and spontaneous-seeming message," she added.[7]

To explore this idea further, I spoke with Susan Lee Colby, the founder and chief creative officer of Grace Creative. Her background includes working with major creative ad agencies like Chiat\Day and BBDO on accounts like Apple and Honda. Colby had a major epiphany at one point in her career. "I realized that as women over 50, we are buying everything. Nobody was talking to us, and if they were talking to us, it was not in the right way. They were talking to us in a very degrading, insulting way."[8] Not only were most advertisers missing their key buyers, but they were also missing an opportunity to appeal to a wider demographic. "Age is actually aspirational for many younger women," Colby said.[9]

This realization led to the birth of Grace Creative more than a decade ago. The company's manifesto states:

> We've worked at big companies, given birth to businesses and families, built our dream homes, downsized, exceeded our goals, reimagined our goals, parented our parents, lost loved ones, retired our egos and refired our dreams, looked at ourselves and seen our mothers, looked at our husbands and thought, "isn't there somewhere you need to be?" Friended, unfriended, and hopefully changed someone's life. You might call it life experience. We call it Grace.[10]

Colby stepped out and launched the business, now with eight full-time employees and a network of creative freelancers all over 50. They have worked with more than twenty client companies.

In the media-buying world, if you dare to suggest that there is an opportunity to target people over 50, it is generally ignored. Deep ingrained thinking and behaviors are hard to change, especially in a world that deals in old constructs. "A part of the issue is that only 1 percent of ad agencies are owned by women of any age, and women over 50 don't get a meaningful voice around the creative table at most agencies," Colby said.[11]

Diane Epstein, a former executive vice president at Dentsu Creative, a global advertising agency, confirmed this, saying, "There is no focus on targeting consumers over 54. Occasionally, there will be a gray-haired person, but that's it."[12]

When one of Epstein's clients wanted to target the 50-plus consumer, Epstein had to go outside the United States to find creative directors to work with for the effort. "Most advertising agencies don't think about figuring out a way to keep experienced professionals. There is no creative voice at 50 at the table," she said.[13]

women over 50 don't get a meaningful voice around the creative table at most agencies

As a result, the messaging and imagery defaults to stereotypical representation of people over 50. We've all seen it. Passive couples walking hand in hand into the sunset, people who are sedentary, tech-phobic, or only focused on their ailments.

Paul Woolmington, a long-time advertising leader and currently CEO at Canvas Worldwide, one of the largest private media buying companies concurs. "The dynamics and economics of the over-50 market is still not being fully recognized in marketing. It's a sad commentary," he said.[14]

Woolmington is one of the few leaders who recognizes what he calls this massive economic powerhouse. It's especially massive when you step back and look at the incredible subsegments in this age group. "The advertising world hasn't been given a contemporary look at this segment by their consumer insights teams, especially the subsets who spend off the Richter scale in categories like housing, automotive, technology, and more. In today's world, brands have the ability to test, learn, and scale new kinds of efforts due to digital capabilities."[15]

According to him, brands are considered contemporary if they have a gay couple or a mixed-race couple in an ad, but even most contemporary brands haven't made the leap to a modern interpretation of what today's 50-plus-year-old might look like. "Unfortunately, a lot of pharmaceutical ads still show stereotypes of people over 50, and they spend a lot of advertising dollars targeting that group. It just reinforces old-fashioned images."[16]

A&E, the cable network, released a major study on the subject in 2022 that included an in-depth look at advertising. In an AI-driven ad audit of twenty thousand television ads in all categories, only one in ten faces were over 50.[17] Another study from CreativeX analyzed more than 126,000 ads across all categories to find that only 4 percent of the people depicted were over 60[18]—even though people over 60 represent 16 percent of the population.

In 2023, global research conducted by Boston Consulting Group's Center for Customer Insight underscored the increasing importance of this expanding group. In the twelve markets they studied, 870 million people from 50 to 70 years old were responsible for 27 percent of spending, around $7 trillion each year in the nine product categories they researched. The study pointed out that mature consumers are willing to spend more money on quality products. The study goes on to reveal various ways marketers need to think about this market segment, noting that while 36 percent of Americans are currently 50 plus, that will grow to 42 percent by 2050. In Japan, it will be 56 percent and in China, 52 percent.[19] This group will only get larger and more impactful in spending power.

The idea of targeting anyone over 54 in an advertising buy is rarely discussed among marketers, unless it is a pharmaceutical brand. Then the idea is to place a commercial on a television network, because the belief is that anyone that age only watches television and isn't active on digital and social media platforms. However, the Boston Consulting Group's study found that around 90 percent of people aged 50–70 use social media platforms a least once a day.[20]

David Sable shared what might be behind this disconnect. "A part of the problem is that media is being bought by younger people who don't really understand what media can accomplish. They focus on programmatic digital buys and use a bunch of dropdown menus to buy the media and watch the analytics," he said.[21]

Like the Boston Consulting Group study, Pew Research reported that consumers over 50 are active on social media platforms from Facebook and YouTube to Pinterest and TikTok.[22] Of the 2.5 billion worldwide users of TikTok, more than 460 million of them are 55 plus. Social media has spawned a "shadow media" universe of older influencers who have disrupted the imagery and messaging that established brands, who continue to live in their old paradigm, are missing. These ageless influencers include Crystal Renee, Nikol Sanchez, Grece Ghanem, and Joan Mac-Donald, as well as Barbara Costello and the Old Gays.

There are now many ways to find more authentic images of people over 50. Getty, Shutterstock, and Adobe have all upgraded their photography selections. The UK-based Centre for Aging Better has a free library showing positive and realistic images of people over 50. The Wallis Annenberg GenSpace group in Los Angeles has created a resource guide for content creators that is useful in all creative circles from advertising to entertainment. To challenge the larger brand and marketing universe, there is now an entire ecosystem being built to address the modern 50-plus world. It's a classic disruption technique.

As Woolmington put it, "The general agency world and brands need to wake up to what is happening."[23]

Emerging Re-Imagineer Marketing Leaders

Fortunately, there is an emerging group of Re-Imagineer marketing leaders who are leading the way with new brand and communication strategies. They include new brands like CADDIS, the eye appliance company that states on its website, "CADDIS is calling bullshit on 50 is the new 40, on the whole fountain of youth illusion, on the many industries that are profiting on vanity and the fear of age, on the concept of 'aging gracefully' and on the notion of raging against the dying of the light."[24]

L'Oréal has also been a pioneer in celebrating age inclusivity, incorporating images of older women in their "Because You're Worth It" campaign. Their advertising approach has incorporated women from Julianna Margulies to Helen Mirren and has been going strong for 40 years.

Global brand Estée Lauder created a campaign in Scandinavia with the then-58-year-old former Danish Prime Minister Helle Thorning-Schmidt called Because of My Age. "This is about changing the conversation for the beauty industry," said Lauder's Kwok.[25] The campaign has appeared in the United Kingdom, Western Europe, the United States, and Canada. It's part of a larger global effort from Estée Lauder that leans into the new longevity. They established the Skin Longevity Institute to create a conversation with consumers of all ages with an emphasis on those who are 50 plus. The content goes beyond product messaging to educate customers about living a longer and healthier life. Taking it one step farther, in 2025, Estée Lauder named 60-year-old model Paulina Prizkova as their brand ambassador.

QVC is another brand that made the strategic decision to lean into their core market in a fresh and innovative way. Like many other brands, they spent a lot of time trying to attract the 18–to–34-year-old segment, until they saw that their best customers were 50 and older.[26] Annette Dunleavy, former vice president of the QVC brand, launched the groundbreaking "Age of Possibility" campaign, celebrating and engaging women over 50. She and her team established the "Quintessential 50," women from 50 to 80 who are changemakers and innovators in their categories. They include makeup artist Mally Roncal, fashion designer Susan Graver, and chef and author Carla Hall. These role models for the new longevity have influenced QVC's communications, social media, and programming.

Other examples of companies adapting their marketing to appeal to older audiences include 50-year-old David Beckham as the face (and body) of the BOSS ONE Bodywear campaign and Prudential Financial's campaign, which highlights a busy mom who has decided to pursue something new after retiring.

Some industry leaders have also highlighted the importance of speaking to older audiences in new ways. Stephanie Fierman, executive vice president of the Association of National Advertisers, is one of the few visionaries who understands what is happening. She and her colleagues have covered the topic of the new 50-plus segment at their industry conferences, podcasts, and committee meetings. Treating this group as the next potential growth market has put them at the forefront of innovative thinking.

Ironically, many other advertising groups continue to have a deaf ear for the topic. It's just another example of the age phobia that continues to exist in the advertising world. When I reached out to one of these groups to make a presentation about the new longevity and how marketers could benefit from it, they responded by asking if I wanted to do a mentoring session with younger professionals. While that's certainly a worthwhile idea, the head of programming completely missed the point.

Of course, the challenges and opportunities that come with marketing to mature consumers is not limited to the United States. There are now more people in the United Kingdom aged over 60 than there are under 18.[27] This group of 15.5 million represents 23 percent of the population and is growing, according to Debbie Marshall, who launched the Silver Marketing Association, a group for connecting and informing businesses that serve the mature market.

When I spoke to her about the issues she sees in this space, she said,

> The UK has many of the same challenges as the US when it comes to marketing to the "silver" demographic. Whilst some sectors have made progress—particularly travel, later-life housing, and finance—there's still a blind spot, largely because the average age of people working in advertising is 28, and you are considered "over the hill" by 35 here. We celebrate ethical age-inclusive marketing, as well as calling out advertisements that could do better.[28]

Changes in the World of Entertainment

While the advertising and marketing worlds are lagging in how they are responding to this new reality, they might take some cues from the entertainment world, which has become aware of the changes in the culture. From shows like *The Golden Bachelor* and *The Golden Bachelorette* to *The Later Daters* on Netflix, programming is shifting in recognition of the dynamic generational change and the vibrancy of older actors. Other examples include *Matlock* with Kathy Bates and *A Man on the Inside* with Ted Danson.

In China, there are at least ten dating shows for older people. In Japan, BS Fuji created a show titled *Nippon no Kaname* (or, *The Heart of Japan*) that was a cross-generational look at addressing the aging population there.

In the United States, the programming "aha" might have started with the series *Grace and Frankie,* starring Jane Fonda and Lily Tomlin, which shattered all expectations, lasting seven seasons and ninety-four episodes. In the *Esquire* article "The Huge, Fast-Growing Audience That Hollywood Is Just Ignoring," Fonda said, "Older women are the fastest-growing demographic in the world. It's a business and if they [Hollywood] want to meet the market, they're going to have to start writing television shows about older women, and they're doing that."[29]

When it comes to movies, the Ed Burns film *Millers in Marriage* boasts a star-studded cast of 50-and-older actors like Julianna Margulies and Patrick Wilson. It explores how three middle-aged couples come to grips with universal questions about marriage and fidelity, professional success and failure, and the challenge of finding a second act.

The trouble is convincing decision makers that movies like this aren't a one-off phenomenon. Hollywood producer Amy Baer cites *The Best Exotic Marigold Hotel* and *Something's Gotta Give* as additional examples of successful films made to appeal to audiences over 50. "But every time there is a success like that, Hollywood executives say, 'WOW, we had no idea that would work.'"[30]

Nevertheless, acting roles, particularly those for women, are beginning to change. A study from UK-based research group AMICA identified Helen Mirren and Judi Dench as the actresses with the most acting credits (forty-six) over the age of 60. Mirren has played everyone from a queen to an assassin. Dench has also played a queen as well as the role of the powerful M, chief of MI6, in seven Bond films.[31] As time goes on, we'll see more of this in television, film, videos, social media, and advertising.

Institutions Have Work to Do

Consumers are way ahead of these institutions that are supposed to reflect the culture. They are looking for the brands, filmmakers, and creatives who get them and represent them in a modern, contemporary way.

In the future, creators in all forms of advertising, entertainment, and imagery will realize that with the huge size and spending power of the 50-plus consumer, they will need to become more age inclusive, but more importantly by using representation that is contemporary and relevant.

They can start by including more 50-and-older creators around the table who can challenge lack of authenticity or unrealistic portrayals. Artificial intelligence is not the answer, as everything it gathers represents old tropes from the past. Real people with real experience will need to lead the way.

The true Re-Imagineers in these industries will enjoy the spoils of the new longevity. The others will have to play a fast game of catch-up.

Consumers are way ahead of these institutions that are supposed to reflect the culture

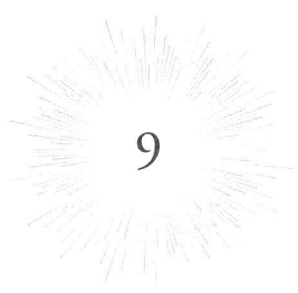

9

The Longevity Travel Era
Comes of Age

If you have been thinking about busting out to do some traveling in the second half of your life, the question is "What are you waiting for?" If you are interested in itineraries that cater to the 50-plus crowd that focus on longevity, wellness, adventure, and health, then your interest is right on one of the biggest global trends in travel. There are now an enormous number of companies ready to cater to your interests, whether you prefer to travel solo, with a partner, or with a group of friends. You can travel to exotic destinations or stay local. The travel industry is reimagining itself in lots of ways to accommodate longevity-focused travelers.

Longevity travel—pursuing longer, healthier lives through curated travel experiences—has become one of the latest trends in the booming wellness tourism industry according to Melissa Biggs Bradley, founder of luxury travel agency Indagare Travel.[1] Modern longevity travel goes beyond traditional spa treatments, combining medical science, holistic wealth, and community engagement.

Add to that the growth in adventure travel and expedition cruises and it is a trend that is here to stay, not just for those over 50 but for younger people who want to pursue wellness in their travel choices and live the longevity life. According to Travel Agent Central, the growth in the number of travelers over 60 is 125 percent since 2020.[2]

In the ROAR forward study of Re-Imagineers, 84 percent of respondents said the number one area they spent their money on was travel, followed by 77 percent whose biggest spend was health and wellness.[3] The confluence of these two areas of interest should continue to drive the massive trend in the wellness and longevity travel industry.

According to the Global Wellness Institute, the global market size for wellness tourism hit $817 billion in 2022 but is projected to grow to $1.3 trillion in 2025. Their definition of the wellness traveler is someone whose trip or destination choice is primarily motivated by wellness, or someone who wants to maintain wellness or participate in wellness experiences while traveling.[4]

In "Defying Convention to Deepen Connections: Booking.com's Nine Predictions for Travel in 2025," the company researched the plans of more than twenty-seven thousand travelers across thirty-three countries.[5] The study revealed that 60 percent of travelers said they are interested in a longevity retreat, especially one that offers revitalization. Of all travelers polled, 56 percent were interested in body vibration, 48 percent in cryotherapy, and 45 percent in stem cell treatment. When they were asked if they would pay for a vacation where the sole purpose was to extend their lifespan and well-being, 58 percent of travelers said yes.[6]

Indagare's 2024 Traveler Sentiment Survey polled around 1,500 of their luxury travel community members and found that two-thirds of respondents will likely plan a wellness-focused trip for their next trip.[7]

Although most people cannot afford it, wellness and longevity travel that caters to the wealthiest is making a big dent in the luxury travel segment. Canyon Ranch in Tucson, Arizona, launched a $20,000 wellness program called LONGEVITY8™. It's four days of working with performance scientists and nutritionists, incorporating integrative medicine, strength, endurance, flexibility, sleep, mental and emotional health, and spiritual wellness. Guests have eighteen one-on-one consultations, fifteen diagnostic tests, and more than two hundred biomarkers measured so that providers can craft a bespoke wellness plan. There are follow-up services and video visits after the experience.[8]

Klara Glowczewska has spent her entire career tracking travel trends. As one of the founding editors of *Condé Nast Traveler*, serving as its editor in chief for nine years, she is now the executive travel editor at *Town & Country* magazine. "There are more and more serious destination spas the world over who are adding longevity elements to their offerings. Hotels are expanding in this era and even cruise ships are getting in the game. They are all responding to a growing consumer interest, which by the way is not just for the over 50+ crowd," she said.[9]

Her examples include the growing number of quasi-medical spa destinations and programs like Seabourn's partnership with integrative medicine guru Andrew Weil and Datu Wellness in Laticastelli, Italy. Lanserhof Sylt, a medical spa in List auf Sylt, Germany, has longevity-enhancing offerings that include brain health and sleep programs as well as INUSpheresis blood-washing therapy, an advanced detoxification process that removes microplastics, heavy metals, and inflammatory fats from the bloodstream. The list goes on, from the famous Clinique La Prairie in Switzerland to Palazzo Fiuggi's Hiking for Longevity program in Italy to Kamalya in Thailand to the Six Senses Kaplankaya longevity wellness program in Turkey. They are all great examples of well-known spas and resorts that are the Re-Imagineer companies in the longevity travel revolution.

In 2025, Estée Lauder joined forces with Hacienda AltaGracia, an Auberge Resort in Costa Rica to launch its first Skin Longevity Institute. Located adjacent to one of the world's five "Blue Zones," they will offer a variety of longevity practices, including elevated skin diagnostics and treatments along with customized programming like mindfulness and hiking in the local mountains of Pérez Zeledón.

According to Biggs Bradley, places like Mii amo in Sedona offer retreats such as "Your Personal Roadmap Towards Longevity" that foster a holistic connection between mental and physical well-being.[10] Other favorites include Chenot Palace Weggis in Switzerland and the SHA Wellness Clinic in Spain.

In late 2024, the lifestyle hospitality company sbe announced their launch of the Estate Hotels & Residences.[11] The locations will focus on functional and preventive medicine through multi-modal diagnostics and vetted therapeutics powered by the Fountain Life Longevity Center. The plan is to open fifteen global hotels and ten urban preventative medicine and longevity centers by 2030.

foster a holistic connection between mental and physical well-being

For the Adventurous Traveler

For many of us, what we now call adventure travel has been a part of our desired travel experience all along, as we pursue ways to stay healthy and active.

In my own adult life, travels with family and friends have shifted to different types of experiences. We still like cultural trips, but we like to mix it up with different kinds of trips and tend to lean towards the adventurous. This passion led to the formation of our adventure travel group of 50-to-75-year-olds. And someday, we'll continue into our 80s and 90s! We pride ourselves on being early adopters in exploring new places that haven't hit the cognoscenti radar yet. For example, in the year 2003, we ventured to Antarctica on a Russian icebreaker called the *Akademik Ioffe*. At the time, luxury Antarctica cruises were a bit of an oxymoron. Companies like Seabourn, Oceania Cruises, and Viking hadn't ventured there yet, but today mainstream travelers are heading to the Blue Continent in droves, becoming de facto adventure travelers. Our group was early in on Namibia and Madagascar, as well as Ethiopia and the Kimberley in Western Australia. The more adventurous the better.

I returned to Antarctica to celebrate my 60th birthday. There, I ran the Antarctica Marathon, capping off my goal to complete seven marathons on seven continents. That was followed by the nine-day hike to Everest Base Camp and the Tenzing Hillary Everest Marathon. (Yes, that exists.)

We're not alone. In the *Wall Street Journal* article "Adventure Travel Is Increasingly Not Just for the Young," adventure travel outfitters reported that the average age of their customers has ticked upwards. For example, Adventure South NZ, a New Zealand-based outfitter, said that the average age of its hiking and biking guests was 55 during the ten years before the pandemic and jumped to 65 directly after.[12]

According to UK company Accor, one of the big trends for British travelers is to combine activities like marathons, triathlons, and other competitive events with exploring new cultures. And they reported a 50 percent uptick in searches for "workout holidays" over the past year.[13]

When I met Tom Hale, the founder of Backroads and a legend in the travel industry, it was a rock star moment. While some people spend their free time browsing through catalogs, magazines, websites, and social media for content about interior design, golf, fashion trends, or fly fishing, I'm addicted to Backroads's catalogs and website. Founded by Hale in 1979, Backroads is the original wellness travel company and the go-to resource if you are interested in hiking, biking, and multi-sport adventures. The company is also an innovator in the explosive trend in longevity and wellness travel for those who want to build on their fitness quotient.

While there are hundreds of destinations to choose from, Backroads has introduced a number of initiatives that target the 50 plus crowd. Hale said the average age of travelers on their hiking and biking trips is 61.[14]

Backroads's Dolce Tempo program is designed for those who want to have a more easygoing experience, as is a new program called Unplugged. While their menu includes trips specifically designed for singles, couples, or families, Hale said their launch of women's adventure trips in 2024 surpassed any kind of rollout they've ever done.[15]

Road Scholar, a nonprofit educational travel organization, is devoted to what I would call "wellness of the brain." Their commitment to educational travel both in person and online has made them one of the premier companies for those over 50 with both wanderlust and curiosity, and they have served six million older adults since their founding in 1975.[16] They have conducted learning adventures across the globe, from art in France to architecture in Prague.

According to James Moses, president of Road Scholar, there are thousands of choices each year, from online programs to immersive in-person learning experiences. Some of them include ship voyages or domestic and global hiking trips. Locations range from Pennsylvania to Tibet, Nepal, and Bhutan. The average age of a first-time participant is around 65, and about two-thirds are women.[17]

Solo travelers make up 25–30 percent of Road Scholar participants, according to Moses. With this in mind, Road Scholar has also created programs for solo travelers only, a great way for individuals to come together for a unique experience. Whether it is a trip to Havana, Buenos Aires, or the great capitals of eastern Europe, the programs create a welcoming community for those who want to travel the world but may not have a partner or friend who shares the same passion. For those clients who are no longer able to travel to physical destinations, Road Scholar has hundreds of online courses and videos that focus on their mission to inspire learning and discovery. "Because people are living so much longer, they are not prepared for the loss of or change in independence, so we now have programs for them," said Moses.[18]

In 2025, Road Scholar also introduced a new series of online lectures focused on what they call the "fourth stage of life," addressing the challenges and opportunities associated with older age. The program, called Age Well, covers health and wellness strategies, emotional well-being and resistance, financial security and planning, social connections and community engagement, and accessibility, technology and independent living.

For the Cruise Lover

The cruise industry has also begun to tap into the longevity and adventure phenomena for travelers. Expedition and exploration are the fastest-growing cruise itineraries. There has been a 71 percent increase in expedition itineraries from 2019 to 2023, a lot of it due to pent-up demand during the COVID years.[19] *AFAR* magazine reported that cruisers are getting more adventurous, including trips into Indonesia's Raja Ampat or to the Kimberley in Western Australia, with side trips to the region's red-rock cliffs, waterfalls, and crocodiles.[20]

Oceania Cruises has wellness discovery tours to learn about different global practices. They also have fitness and training programs from functional stretching to vinyasa yoga, and their cuisine is based in health and wellness. Their Aquamar Spa + Vitality Center includes traditional spa treatments but also pain management programs and a Chinese herbal medical consultation, as well as medi-spa procedures. So passengers have many options to learn more about longevity practices for a healthier and longer life. Oceania partnered with Condé Nast Traveler to curate itineraries for 2025 and 2026 that included a hike to the Ten Thousand Buddhas Monastery, a trek to Mount Aksla in Norway, and more off-ship excursions.

Storylines Cruises plans to take it to another level in 2028 by launching a luxury residential community at sea. In this case, you literally move onto the ship after purchasing a shipboard apartment: It's a floating city of 530 residences, each costing between $2 million and $8 million. The owners will circumnavigate the world for three and a half years, followed by a different course for the next three and a half years. Alister Punton, founder and CEO of Storylines and a travel Re-Imagineer, explained, "The ship called MV *Narrative* will have one of the largest wellness and longevity centers in the world, a ten-thousand-square-foot space devoted to helping our residents live a longer, happier, and healthier life."[21]

In partnership with EnerChanges Health Clinic based in Vancouver, Canada, the plan is to merge world travel with cutting-edge healthcare. Services overseen by Dr. Brian Martin, chief health officer, will include advanced functional testing as well as bioidentical hormone replacement therapy, stem cell therapy, human growth hormones, peptides, and more. "Aside from the most up-to-date longevity care technology, processes and protocols, we'll also have traditional spa treatments, fitness, and open-air sports decks," said Punton.[22]

Once, stereotypical cruise passengers might have lounged by the pool all day and indulged in artery-clogging food every night. Now, the new wave of wellness travelers have some oceangoing options that appeal to their style. Whether they're offering more thrilling adventures, a focus on day-to-day wellness, or longevity treatments on board, these companies are reimagining what cruises can look like for older travelers.

For the Cost-Conscious Traveler

While longevity travel might seem only for the wealthy, there are many other choices that don't have to cost thousands of dollars. Traveling to a place in the United States or just across town is a way for everyone to tap into the longevity phenomena. The YO1 Longevity & Health Resorts in the Catskills in New York is one of many examples. Others include Castle Hot Springs in Morristown, Arizona, Three Forks Ranch in Savery, Wyoming, and the Wiawaka Holiday House in Lake George, New York. While these are more affordable than high-end luxury destinations, there may be some people who cannot afford them but still want to tap into a longevity experience.

Cities and local communities offer programs, many of them free, that can help put you on a journey of wellness and longevity without spending any money on travel, except for transportation across town! The Bridge to Wellness program sponsored by the City of Duluth, Minnesota, offers health fairs and webinars. The Healthy Lifestyle Institute at the University of Pittsburgh provides activity classes and wellness consultation. The Health Sciences Center Wellness program at the University of New Mexico and the Kripalu Center for Yoga & Health also have programs and workshops for longevity health.

The City of Los Angeles Parks Department of Recreation offers yoga in Griffith Park, and New York City's Healthy NYC program and the Blue Zones project are examples of city-sponsored longevity programs. The Blue Zones project is transforming towns across North America to help people live longer with a higher quality of life. They currently operate in seventy-five communities, bringing together local stakeholders and international well-being experts to introduce evidence-based programs to measurably improve well-being.

Pursue Your Longevity-Inspired Travel Dreams

Longevity-inspired travel is here to stay, and travel industry Re-Imagineers are redefining their offerings in new and imaginative ways. Whether you prefer your travel experience to involve a luxury spa, an exciting adventure, a relaxing cruise, or something a little simpler, there is now a way to plug in to a wellness and longevity destination that will help you start or build on your healthy lifestyle. Adventure awaits you, and the options are going to continue to grow in the years ahead.

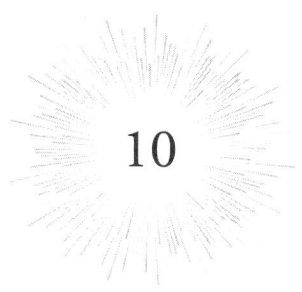

10

The New Longevity Medicine and Its Impact on All of Us

When I got to the Stanford campus to meet with Ronjon Nag, I have to admit that I was very intimidated by the idea of interviewing him. Aside from his academic credentials, which include a PhD in engineering from Cambridge, a postdoctoral fellowship at Stanford, and a master's degree in management science from the MIT Sloan School of Management, he has a long list of accomplishments.[1] He is an adjunct professor in genetics at the Stanford School of Medicine and the founder and president of R42 Group, a family office and venture group which invests in AI, biotechnology, and science. The group has invested in more than a hundred AI biotech companies, according to Nag. I should also mention that he has been involved in a long list of many firsts, including the first continuous blood pressure wearable (GT Cardio, 2019) and the first neural network artificial intelligence system in the cloud (Ersatz Labs, 2014).

Nag was warm and welcoming and unexpectedly down to earth. We chatted about his many experiences and his passion for learning and teaching. We found common ground as fellow marathoners. He then told me about his newest focus, a company that he founded called Agemica and the "moonshot" project to develop a vaccine to slow down the aging process. "Our goal is not to fix aging, but to add another twenty years or more to life," he explained. "Artificial intelligence can help to extend the healthy lifespan of humans."[2]

Agemica is working on developing drug combinations that reduce biological age and prevent the diseases of aging. According to Nag, in the future, we won't do drug trials anymore but go right to AI-proven drug solutions. Bringing anti-aging therapies to market fast is the goal. A great example of how this can work is when Moderna used artificial intelligence tools to create the mRNA vaccine for COVID and get it to market in a couple of months versus spending years in clinical trials. As of 2025, Agemica's technology had already rediscovered standards of care for seventeen cancer areas that he believes is the pathway to bigger success.

Nag explained that an AI-driven approach will help identify the root causes of aging and slow down cardiovascular disease and neurodegeneration. I realized that his work, and the work of so many others, is leading us into a future that none of us can truly understand yet. When I asked him if I needed to follow up on any of my notes, he suggested that I just reach out to his AI assistant, who would be able to answer any questions I might have about his work.

As Dorothy said, "We're not in Kansas anymore!"

The Re-Imagineers of Longevity Medicine

As I set out to learn more about what is happening in the world of medicine and how technology will drive the longevity phenomenon, it became clear that this is one of the most exciting times in history. New medical breakthroughs will not only revolutionize our lifespan and health span but potentially lead to pushing out life expectancies to 100 or more in a short period of time, all fueled by the AI revolution.

this is one of the most exciting times in history

During my research for this chapter, it also became clear that this topic could be a book unto itself. I could have easily spoken to hundreds of individuals around the world who are engaged in longevity medicine and all of its dimensions. Although the following people represent only a small portion of that larger number, each is engaged in particularly interesting, useful work that has the potential to change the process of aging forever.

Eric Verdin, Buck Institute for Research on Aging

Eric Verdin has served as the president and CEO of the Buck Institute for Research on Aging since 2016. Belgian-born Verdin earned a doctorate of medicine from the University of Liege, then trained at Harvard Medical School and has held faculty positions at the National Institutes of Health, the Picower Institute for Medical Research, the Gladstone Institute, and the University of California, San Francisco.[3] (At the start of our Zoom call, I shared my enthusiasm for a recent visit to Antwerp, not far from his hometown of Liege.)

The Buck Institute researches aging and ways to extend healthy years of life. Founded in 1999, it was the world's first organization to study intervention into the aging process. Since Verdin has joined, the Institute has grown to three hundred people and from a budget of $32 million to $65 million today. His vision is to double it again in the next ten to fifteen years to accelerate their work. "The goal is not to double it for the sake of doubling it, but really to add to this whole new dimension of human health," he explained.[4]

The Buck Institute has been a consistent trailblazer in the study of aging. It was there that the term *geroscience* was coined. The idea is that aging is a major risk factor for chronic diseases. The goal is to identify the drivers of the aging process. "The promise of geroscience is that by targeting aging itself and its pathways, we can suppress the development of diseases such as the many forms of cancer, heart disease, osteoporosis, neurodegeneration (Parkinson's and Alzheimer's disease) that are all linked to the aging process" said Verdin.[5]

One step that Verdin is leading to reimagine Buck's future has been the establishment of the Center for Human Healthspan, a partnership with Phenome Health to translate innovative new science-of-aging approaches from new drug compounds and preclinical models to computational technologies and algorithms to clinical practice. "We've made two very visible recruitments in this effort. One of them is Lee Hood, a legend in biology. He's a member of all three National Academies and has won every prize except the Nobel Prize. He's an incredibly visionary scientist who was behind the invention of the first DNA sequencing machine that led to the Human Genome Project," explained Verdin.[6]

The other exciting hire at Buck was Dr. Nathan Price, who is a professor and codirector of the Center and coauthored the bestselling book *The Age of Scientific Wellness* with Hood. Like Hood, he has a long list of accomplishments, including his current role of chief scientific officer of Thorne, a healthy aging company. According to Verdin, Hood and Price created an AI platform that can analyze huge amounts of data and aid the Buck Institute in making discoveries that can improve human health and increase longevity. "There is also a whole new series of technologies called Omics that allow us to measure tens of thousands of variables in one single measurement. They are proteomics, metabolomics, and transcriptomics. They are currently research tools, but we predict in the future they will become clinical tools, especially to assess human health," he explained.[7]

I asked him what an outcome might be should this become a new part of the medical landscape. "If you go to see a doctor right now, you will have a blood panel with about a hundred values, but our biology is much more complex. An example would be using proteomics as a tool. We have twenty-five thousand different proteins, and proteomics allows us to quantify many of them very precisely in one sample. Using AI, we will get a much deeper understanding of our individual self."[8]

The technology can also be used in a predictive manner. Imagine a world where you go to a doctor at the age of 30 or 35 and the doctor can identify your susceptibility to cancer or heart disease based on data analysis. According to Verdin, identifying this early is a way to revert the disease process at a stage where it's much more primitive and simpler. He added that in the future of medicine, doctors will be able to

Imagine a world where you go to a doctor at the age of 30 or 35 and the doctor can identify your susceptibility to cancer or heart disease based on data analysis

increase the resolution of a clinical diagnosis. Preliminary data indicates that a disease like type 2 diabetes, which is diagnosed once your blood sugar goes over a certain limit, actually represents different diseases with different specific interventions. That new frontier of medicine is called *precision medicine*, a treatment that is for your individual biology.

Buck is one of the leading organizations to focus on the future of healthy aging through personalized, data-driven science. In simple terms, healthcare providers in the future will be able to assess individual biological markers, clinical data of social determinants of health, and digital measures of environmental exposures and behaviors (assessed through wearables) to have a deep, holistic understanding of the individual.

With AI capabilities, how you are treated for a disease will be different than how I am treated for the same disease based on our individual profiles, hence the term precision medicine. This customization of healthcare is already here and can be used in both treatments and preventative care. This breakthrough is a major step in the world of longevity medicine and expanding our individual healthy lifespans.

Mark Lachs, Cornell Center for Aging Research and Clinical Care

Dr. Mark Lachs, MD, MPH, is the Irene and Roy Psaty Distinguished Professor of Medicine at the Weill Cornell Medical College in New York and the first director of the Cornell Center for Aging Research and Clinical Care (CARCC), among many other accomplishments. Long engaged in longevity medicine and science as a trained geriatrician, Lachs said, "In the 1950s, we studied organs, in the '60s cells, and in the '70s organelles, which is machinery within cells. Fast forward and we are now studying humans at the molecular and even submolecular level. This is all leading to the new discoveries in longevity that is transforming medicine."[9]

At this fine level, researchers can look for biologic "hallmarks of aging." One example is DNA methylation, which is the tendency for a small carbon-hydrogen molecule to bind to DNA at faster and faster rates as we age. Another is telomere shortening. Telomeres, Lachs explained, "protect the ends of chromosomes from becoming frayed or tangled when cells divide. With each division, telomeres become shorter and shorter, and ultimately too short to divide. As a result we become more vulnerable to age-related diseases.[10]

Why is it important to identify these hallmarks of aging? Two reasons: First, they are logical targets for drug or behavioral interventions that can slow these processes. Second, they can be seen as biological "aging clocks"; when healthcare providers administer a new drug or behavioral intervention (like more exercise or better sleep) they can biologically measure its impact in addition to the subjective sense of well-being in the person they're treating.

According to Lachs, aging is the major risk factor for the onset of all chronic diseases—cancer, heart disease, arthritis, you name it. Yet we target individual diseases instead of the biology of aging itself. But the world is changing, which is why geroscience is now the most exciting field of biology and attracting hoards of young scientists.

aging is the major risk factor for the onset of all chronic diseases

While Lachs concurs that the future of all medicine is precision medicine, he also believes that longevity will be influenced by non-medical issues like environment, relationships, hope, meaning, purpose, and work. (Lachs also wants to see how changes in those factors influence the biological clock.)

What about a pill that can help on the biological front? Can that help us live longer? There is much that is being written about metformin, rapamycin, and even Ozempic, Wegovy, and Mounjaro as potential drugs to influence the aging process. Dozens more are in development. For example, there is a class of drugs called senolytics that target and eliminate senescent cells, those cells that no longer work well in our bodies. Some of these drugs include fisetin and reseveratrol. "These are not drugs that reverse aging or are a cure for aging, but might delay the aging process. Imagine delaying the diagnosis of dementia by a decade," said Lachs."[11]

At first glance, it may not sound like a breakthrough. But in fact, it would delay or avoid immeasurable suffering to patients and families and save the US economy billions of dollars, as people could retain functional abilities to the very end of life.

Nir Barzilai, Albert Einstein College of Medicine

Dr. Nir Barzilai is known for his study of centenarians at the Albert Einstein College of Medicine in New York.[12] He is one of the proponents of the emergence of these new drugs. His project TAME (Targeting Aging with METformin) is to study if the drug can delay the onset of age-related diseases, including cancer, cardiovascular disease, and more. Sponsored by the American Federation for Aging Research (AFAR) and the National Institute on Aging, the study will enroll three thousand people between the ages of 65 and 79 for a six-year trial.

Barzilai and his coauthor Michael Leone also published a study online in February 2024, *Evaluating Possible Anti-Aging Drugs*, which explores a long list of potential solutions.[13] There's only one big hitch when it comes to drugs for aging: The FDA will not currently approve a drug with an indication of preventing aging.

Thomas Rando, UCLA, the American Federation for Aging

In September 2024 I asked Dr. Thomas Rando about the FDA's refusal to approve anti-aging drugs. Rando is a professor of neurology and molecular, cell, and developmental biology at UCLA and the president of the American Federation for Aging.

He responded, "The main reason for the FDA issue is that we don't have a good measure of aging except for death. No clinical trials are going to treat you until you die, and that would be too expensive and may take decades. The solution? A blood test like cholesterol for statins where you can say, 'This drug is actually working because it is slowing down aging.'"[14]

The current data for both metformin and rapamycin comes from animal trials, although there is some epidemiologic data that is promising. As mentioned in chapter 1, metformin has been shown to reduce the harmful effects of senescent cells and rapamycin is an mTOR inhibitor that can delay the development of cellular senescence.

"In Scandinavia, there is a study showing that if you compare how long people lived with diabetes with metformin or without metformin, those on metformin lived longer. But that is not a clinical trial, per se," said Rando.[15] While none of these drugs have been proven to delay aging in humans, they present interesting implications for the future and possibility for further breakthroughs in this area of science.

Jennifer Garrison, Buck Institute for Research on Aging, ProductiveHealth.org

Dr. Jennifer Garrison, assistant professor and codirector of the Center for Healthy Aging in Women at the Buck Institute for Research on Aging until mid 2025 and the cofounder and executive director of ProductiveHealth.org, is one of the important global female voices on longevity.[16] Her work to fundamentally transform women's health by optimizing ovarian function across female lifespan won first place at the XPRIZE Global Visioneering Conclave. In 2025, she competed to win the XPRIZE itself in the health domain.

Garrison helped start the Center for Healthy Aging in Women at Buck in 2019. It's the first center in the world to focus on the idea that female reproductive organs might have a real impact on longevity in the rest of the body. She has also created a global consortium to build the ecosystem of scientists and clinicians who, along with funders, entrepreneurs, and policymakers, are dedicated to understanding this better.

"We used to call it the Center and Global Consortium for Reproductive Longevity and Equality, but we rebranded to the Center for Healthy Aging in Women and the Productive Health Global Consortium, removing the word 'reproductive' so that we are not pigeonholing all of women's health through the lens of fertility," she explained.[17]

A neuroscientist by training, Garrison believes reframing women's health through the lens of ovarian function is really the breakthrough idea. She explained, "Ovaries profoundly impact health and health span. They are sitting at the center of a really complex signaling network and communicate with nearly every organ in a woman's body. They talk to bone and brain and heart and liver and the list goes on."[18] While the ovaries play a significant role in a woman's body from puberty through fertility and menopause, non-functioning ovaries can lead to many health issues from cardiovascular disease to stroke and other conditions. Garrison's work is focused on the importance of maintaining healthy ovaries throughout a woman's life.

"The problem that we have is that there's a huge disparity in research around women's health. There is an enormous data gap because of a huge funding gap. With regard to understanding ovarian aging, the funding has been less than 0.1 percent, yet this impacts half the population" she said.[19]

The consortium she has spearheaded is meant to fund grants to scientists all over the world to study what's driving ovarian aging. The first grants were made in 2020 and there has already been enormous progress, including large-scale omics datasets to build on the work. They initiated the world's first global conference on the topic to share findings, and more than fifty papers have been published as a result of the funding. The "return on philanthropy" includes discovery of a novel hormone that builds bone, as well as the first-ever clinical trial that's looking at rapamycin as a prevention for ovarian aging.

In the field of longevity medicine, Garrison has emerged as one of the leaders. As she and her colleagues integrate AI functionality into their work, the breakthrough findings will have an enormous impact in women's health for the current and next generations.

Longevity Health in Singapore

This isn't the first time in this book that I've mentioned longevity efforts in Singapore, and it won't be the last. This is because Singapore is far ahead of most countries when it comes to understanding and acting on many aspects of longevity. Their population has one of the highest life expectancies in the world at 84 years, according to Worldometer.[20]

When I attended the Milken Institute Asia Summit in 2024, I listened with great awe to Esther Krofah, executive vice president of Milken Institute Health, interview Ong Ye Kung, the minister of health for Singapore, about Healthier SG (Healthier Singapore). "Healthier SG is a national initiative to change human behavior at the population level. It is also a focus on preventative care," explained Ong.[21] A platform for innovation, it allows Singaporeans to take more direct control of their health. As of early 2025, more than one million have registered on the platform, nearly 20 percent of the country's population.[22] By enrolling with a family doctor, the individual can establish a holistic approach to health that includes prompts for various tests and merchant vouchers for fulfilling certain exercise goals via the National Steps Challenge.

The White Paper on Healthier SG published in 2022 outlines multiple key features of the program:

- incentives for residents to pay attention to their health through fully subsidized nationally recognized screenings and vaccinations, as well as incentives for drug costs and more
- twelve care protocols to guide family doctors on how to provide holistic care

- the option for Singaporeans to connect to a wide range of activities via community agencies such as Sport Singapore and the Health Promotion Board as ways to adopt healthier lifestyles
- the use of technology to have a digitally enabled health plan to access information in a safe environment[23]

Since one in four Singaporeans is expected to be age 65 or above by 2030, Ong and his team are a collection of Re-Imagineers who are rethinking how to create a healthier population for the future.[24] Singapore is committed to the longevity phenomena in this countrywide initiative.

While I was in Singapore, I met Dr. Andrea Maier from the National University of Singapore (NUS). Maier is a professor of medicine, but is also the founding president of the Healthy Longevity Medicine Society, an international medical group that promotes the highest standards of clinical practice to optimize health span by targeting the aging process across the lifespan.[25] The Department of Health, Abu Dhabi, was their first global partner in defining healthy longevity medicine, according to Maier, and they're in conversations with different ministries to work on the scope and practice for other countries too. Maier is also the founder of Chi Longevity, a global center of excellence for evidence-based biological age discovery and reversal that works to incorporate the latest technology into their clinics. In 2024, they opened their first partnership with the Four Seasons hotel in Singapore and have four other global locations in the works. Maier described the work they do at Chi:

> For our members, we are doing clinical testing from heart to soul. It includes the entire suite of data gathering, from genome epigenetic tests, microbiomes, and other biomarkers, as well as testing hormones, cognition, and psychological assessments. We can track our clients 24/7, as we have everything integrated and are agnostic to their devices, whether it is a Garmin or WHOOP. It allows us to deliver on what we call precision geromedicine.[26]

Chi is one example of the rise of longevity clinics around the world. Others include Fountain Life and Next Health. They are operating in major cities like New York, Dallas, Houston, and Miami, with more to come. The Sheba Longevity Center in Tel Aviv, Israel, and the Mayo Clinic Healthy Living Program in the United States are also bringing longevity medicine to the masses. The opportunities in this space are almost endless, especially when they are aided by technology and artificial intelligence. It is exciting to imagine the longevity-related discoveries that facilities like Chi will make in the coming years.

Longer, Healthier Lives

In researching this book, it became apparent to me that the field of medicine is reimagining ways we will live longer, healthier lives for generations to come. The developments are happening at such an astounding pace that I'm convinced that living to 100 or older will become normalized, certainly for many babies who are being born today. The challenge we all face on a global level is how we make sure the miracles of medicine that facilitate longevity are not just available to the wealthy, but are democratized and widespread for all human beings on the planet. It's a tall order, but the medical professionals I talked to are devoted to this idea. Their work as Re-Imagineers is helping us find the pathways to the true definition of longevity, which means longer, healthier lives in mind, body, and spirit for everyone.

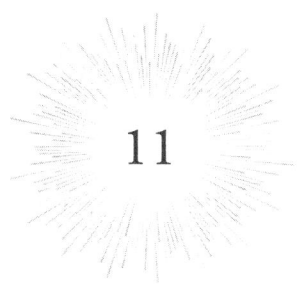

11

The Intersection of Medicine, Health, and Technology: It's Here

As the field of longevity medicine and the future of aging contin-ues to grow, it is being fueled by a cadre of Re-Imagineers that includes doctors, technologists, investors, and founders of longevity clinics, several of which we learned about in the previous chapter. These Re-Imagineers have developed numerous devices and epigenetic tests that allow us to measure our biomarkers and track our health in ways that just ten years ago would have seemed impossible. The development in these sectors is moving at such a rapid pace that by the time this book has reached you, there will have been more progress on this front that I haven't been able to capture. Most of my conversations took place at the end of 2024 and the first half of 2025, but everyone I spoke with assured me that by 2026, there would be much more to talk about with more discoveries, a lot of it being enabled by new AI tools.

Investing in Longevity

One of my go-to sources to get an understanding of the overall longevity investment landscape is Phil Newman, founder and CEO of Longev-ity.Technology and founder of First Longevity, which brings together international investors and longevity start-ups. Newman holds a Lon-gevity Investors Conference every year that helps put shape around this fast-growing, chaotic segment. Like any sector that is still forming, there are multiple moving parts that can create confusion, as well as opportunity.

The numbers from the 2024 conference showed that 2024 total financing in the longevity sector reached $8.4 billion across 331 deals.[1] That includes a broad range of twenty-five longevity domains from diagnostics to cellular re-programming to longevity clinics that are all expanding exponentially. Newman also tracks the number of longevity deals and where the money is going to by quarter and by year, as well as keeping tabs on 1,300 longevity companies, including those involved in longevity neuropharma, longevity discovery platforms, and the diagnostics space.[2]

Many companies, such as those discussed in the previous chapter, are already involved in the longevity business in some form, but the potential for growth in this space is enormous. As a result, it's no surprise that venture capital, including longevity funds, is actively looking for ways to get in on the ground floor or fuel next-stage growth. Some of the major funds include Juvenescence, which focuses on developing therapies to increase human longevity; Apollo Health Ventures; and the Longevity Fund, which was founded in 2011 by Laura Deming and supports start-ups that develop therapies and technologies to combat aging and extend healthy human lifespan.

the potential for growth in this space is enormous

Another important longevity fund is Primetime Partners, which has invested in nearly forty companies.[3] According to cofounder Abby Levy, Primetime Partners is interested in companies that are focused on the data and distribution infrastructure to help bring innovation to life in the field of longevity. "One of the themes we are interested in is pharmacogenomics. With precision polypharmacy, we should be able to combine your genetics and your bloodmarkers to get a better recommendation on which pharmaceuticals or supplements are right for you individually," Levy explained.[4]

In order to put some rigor around the number of new companies and initiatives in the space, Phil Newman has developed what he calls the ten levels that define longevity. It's a road map to understanding the various components of the sector, both present and future.

Newman's first five levels are for what he calls "longevity now" companies, as opposed to those that are more in the concept or development phase.[5] These levels are great guideposts for investors who might be interested in getting investing in longevity. Newman's goal is to provide guidance on what is happening in this fast-moving sector, giving insights, data, and perspective. As he explains in his twelve-minute "Ten Levels of Longevity" lecture on YouTube, no one level is more important than the other, but rather they identify different investment opportunities within existing or emerging sectors of longevity.

Level one is core lifestyle management for longevity, to prevent aging diseases: this includes diet, sleep, exercise, alcohol intake, smoking, stress, and so on. Companies that make wearable technology like WHOOP, Oura, and others are emerging in this area as people track their sleep patterns, heart and respiratory rates, and more. The investment opportunity that Newman touts is AI-supported hyper-personalization for the individual within the wearable space or the emergence of apps that allow you to photograph your food to get automatic calorie and protein intake numbers. This is one area for investors to think about.

Level two is consumer diagnostics, which is the use of biological samples, digital information, and AI to identify opportunities for both clinical and lifestyle interventions to improve health span. Multiomics platforms seek to extend science into consumer products. For investing, Newman recommends companies that bridge mainstream clinical practice and aging biotech research. However, there is still a lot of work that needs to be done to standardize testing of the biomarkers of aging, as one test may produce different results than another one. As Newman told me, "A surrogate age marker that everyone accepts has to be developed, since we can't wait thirty or forty years for the results [of the the tests]."[6]

Level three is dietary supplements to enhance metabolism and replace cellular function lost with the progression of age. There are many products in the marketplace, but not enough human evidence to support serious medical claims, according to Newman. The trend is companies combining longevity molecules into new dietary and cosmetic products. Companies using AI to identify unique GRAS (generally recognized as safe) molecules can tap into this trend. "Brands like Tru Niagen have a lot of clinical evidence behind them, as does MitoQ, a mitochondrial supplement for health span," said Newman.[7]

Level four is professional clinical services for longevity, where people can seek a diagnosis of health and aging biomarkers, clinical guidance on lifestyle and diet, and therapeutic interventions to mitigate the progression of age. This fast-growing investment opportunity (Newman's group tracks 263 companies at this level) includes Chi Longevity in Singapore, Next Health, Fountain Life, and many more.

Level five is clinical interventions that manage the symptoms of diagnosed aging diseases. This is the healthcare system, but as it stands now it's an exciting new dimension for longevity investors. At this level you'll find AI companies that focus on aging drivers that can positively affect aging diseases. That could include pre-clinical companies capable of partnering with pharma business development teams, as an example. "There are now companies that are moving into understanding the hallmarks of aging. They are working on those drivers that are at a metabolic and cellular level in the body. If they can understand and control these pathways, it will create a new approach to stopping a disease in the first place," said Newman.[8]

Levels six through ten are companies in development. There is work being done and investments to support it. This includes diabetes prevention and weight loss therapeutics like Ozempic and Wegovy, which may extend longevity, but the data isn't there yet. According to Newman, there are thirty-five companies focused on ways to reverse aging.

The development of the longevity industry, as outlined by Newman, is attracting different kinds of investors who have become interested in the space. Dr. Peter H. Diamandis, who is best known as the founder and chairman of XPRIZE, made a blog post titled "Billionaires Investing in Longevity." In it, he identifies companies that have recently been founded by billionaires around the world to conduct longevity-related medical and technological research. One such example is Altos, launched in 2022 by Jeff Bezos and Yuri Milner with $3 billion in funding. Altos's mission is to restore cell health and resilience through cellular rejuvenation programming, with the ultimate goal of reversing disease, injury, and age-related disabilities. Another is

NewLimit, cofounded by Coinbase CEO Brian Armstrong and venture capitalist Blake Byers, with a unique approach in the development of epigenetic reprogramming medicines. Retro Bio has the goal of extending human health span by ten years.[9]

Another company, Hevolution Foundation, was launched in 2021 and is a global nonprofit organization that provides grants to incentivize independent research and entrepreneurship in the emerging field of health span science. Headquartered in Riyadh, Saudi Arabia, the organization has the vision to make an extended healthy lifespan a possibility for all humanity through new treatments, faster drug development, increased accessibility to therapeutics, and more. Their primary investment focus is on companies that target the root cause of aging.

As Newman looks farther into the future, he is tracking companies and investors that are also looking at the ability to regenerate the whole human organism or surpass traditional organ replacement through 3D bio-printing, xenotransplantation, or lab-grown organs.[10] To reach far into the future, he notes that companies are emerging that specialize in research into the preservation of the body and/or consciousness of people facing a deadly disease. In theory, this would enable the body or consciousness to be held in some type of storage until drugs or therapeutics were developed to treat the disease, at which point the person would be brought back to life for the treatments and to presumably live a very long life.

That may seem like a science-fictional stretch, but what is certain is that this is all an industry in motion. New uses of AI will emerge, companies will merge and be acquired, and new companies will be born. The players in these areas will continue to grow, and global investment will help them build their future.

The Impact of Technology on Longevity Medicine

Dr. David Luu, the French board-certified surgeon, has become a Re-Imagineer in longevity medicine. He launched Longevity Docs, the first network dedicated to physicians pioneering precision and evidence-based practices in the field.[11] What started as a WhatsApp group led to a Slack channel, which then led to a tech platform to help educate doctors of all specialties in the fast-emerging field of longevity medicine.

With hundreds of doctors from around the globe as part of his group, Luu sponsors in-person gatherings and hosted the first global meeting of his group in Cannes in 2025.

When I spoke with Luu in December 2024, he remarked on the rapid changes that medicine has been undergoing due to advances in technology and AI capabilities: "We are going to have the best understanding of complex human biology that we have ever had."[12] However, he noted that there was still considerable work that needed to be done before the data can be used effectively, because "most doctors have not been trained in AI precision diagnostic personalized medicine and biotechnology, but all of that will have to change."[13]

According to Luu, more and more people are accessing health content through leaders in the space, like Andrew Huberman, as well as online and in the media. As people learn about metformin and wearables and epigenetic testing, they are turning to their doctors to see if pursuing any of these paths is right for them. The goal of Longevity Docs is to help every doctor become a part of the growing conversation and convey the right kind of advice and guidance. "In the conversations among our doctor members, it might go from rapamycin to new technology applications, or how peptides like Ozempic have shown some promising results on longevity factors," he said.[14]

He acknowledges that his group also has to wade through a lot of hype around products that people want to sell as longevity enhancers without any true data to support the claims. Luu's goal is to bring more doctors into the longevity field by creating a community that shares policies, approaches, and medical knowledge and conducts collaborative research on the subject. His vision over the next thirty years is for hospital systems, research organizations, and medical schools to integrate longevity medicine into their everyday practices, so that it becomes a mainstay approach for every individual, not just those who can afford access to cutting-edge healthcare practices.

Across the globe, scientists and doctors are finding new ways to utilize technology to improve health spans and care in the era of longevity. Wendy Chapman earned a PhD from the University of Utah in medical informatics with a research focus in natural language processing, and she was most recently the director of the Centre for Digital Transformation of Health at the University of Melbourne in Australia.[15] When we spoke in December 2024, she told me that one of her areas of interest is finding digital solutions within the healthcare system, in particular for people in rural or other areas that have reduced access to traditional healthcare. "An example might be if you have a remote monitor for a pulse oximeter and are having a telehealth visit with your primary care doctor, how do you bring that data to the visit in a way that is actionable and understandable," she explained.[16]

Chapman's work explores ways in which doctors can incorporate digital solutions into their everyday work, especially with the advent of AI applications. A good example being AI-enabled scribes that capture the conversation a doctor is having with a patient, versus having to type it into a laptop. With all of the digital tools, there is still a question of accuracy, safety, and integration into electronic medical records, but Chapman's center imagines a future where the relationship between clinician and patient is guided by clinical data and enabled by digital health technologies that create a connected system. All the solutions will lead to better healthcare outcomes for individuals and their healthy longevity.

Dr. Jennifer Schrack is a professor and director of the Center on Aging and Health at Johns Hopkins University.[17] An epidemiologist, she is focused on the intersection of movement and healthcare as we age, integrating new forms of technology into her work. Along with Dr. Vicki Freedman from the University of Michigan, she also oversees the National Health and Aging Trends Study and other projects to explore many topics, including how changes in movement with aging affects physical and cognitive functioning later in life.

During a Zoom call in December 2024, she told me, "My personal scientific interest is the idea of digital health and understanding different signals from different types of devices that we wear that can tell us about brain, physical, and sensory health. These devices are monitoring us 24/7 in an extreme level of detail."[18] These research-grade devices collect patterns of data that are observed by Schrack, engineers, biostatisticians, and others with the goal of early detection of health issues to improve longevity. "If we can recognize changes in heart rhythms, changes in movement, sleep patterns, and other indicators of poor health, we can start treating it more effectively," said Schrack.[19]

Her work is done using large cohorts of individuals, and the analysis of the data spans the schools of public health, medicine, and nursing with the goal of pushing cutting-edge research so that practitioners can use it to improve the lives of older adults, particularly as the population ages. "The idea is to keep people healthy for longer, so they don't need a lot of care from others as they age," she said.[20]

As the vice president of Digital Health at the Consumer Technology Association (CTA) and producer of the yearly CES show in Las Vegas, René Quashie's focus is on all things digital health. As part of the Digital Health Summit, the AgeTech Pavilion at CES showcases new innovative technologies that consumers can use, particularly for their individual health needs. The ongoing theme for healthcare at CES is "the future of health," with topics including AI, digital therapeutics, genomics, wearables, women's health, and workforce issues, according to Quashie.[21] Most recently, he has seen two major trends emerge: products geared toward sleep and products for hearing health, especially since the FDA made hearing aids available over the counter.

In my conversation with Quashie, he explained that most of these products now come with AI applications that enable people to monitor their own health. He also noted that new products are frequently being released within this space: "There are a lot more next-gen wearables, too, things like smart mirrors that have advanced sensor tech for personalized metrics just by standing there. The French company Withings is one of the innovators in that area."[22]

The home healthcare movement will gather data through medical devices, patient monitoring systems, and other smart home products, aided by AI, and deliver it to a primary care physician for analysis, according to him. The home as high-tech health hub is a transformative trend within the wellness real estate sector, now worth $398 billion and forecast to grow to $887.5 billion by 2027.[23] According to Quashie, CTA is also deeply engaged in working on many of the standards of these products.[24] They've published more than thirty digital health–related standards on everything from sleep to step calculators to cardiac devices, bringing some rigor to these fast-growing categories. They've also developed a standard for the technical measurements of hearing aids (the standard was incorporated into the FDA's final over-the-counter hearing aid regulations published in 2022) and have started a standards group on women's health topics from menopause to cardiac and lung health. The expansion of genomics and personalized medicine driven by technology is another big trend that Quashie sees, but like many, he is concerned if this will be available to everyone at all socioeconomics levels: "While people want to take control of their health, cost is a huge factor. In one of our studies, 53 percent said that they would only use health-related technology if it was free or covered by insurance."[25] The other factor he identifies is today's older people are not digital natives, so there is an adoption issue with regard to new tech products: "Millennials have the highest rate of tech adoption and ownership in the United States, according to our study. They are very comfortable with technology, and they will be very different tech savvy 60-, 70-, and 80-year-olds someday."[26]

At the forefront of the longevity revolution, CTA is also contemplating the idea of longevity events and programming, capturing more of the products, services, and data that will enable many people to live longer and healthier lives. While new technologies are emerging at a rapid pace, the question is how people keep up with new developments, regardless of their age.

While people want to take control of their health, cost is a huge factor

Dr. Sara Czaja, PhD, a professor at Weill Cornell Medicine in New York and the director of the Center on Aging and Behavioral Research, has spent years at the intersection of technology and longevity.[27] Her research includes looking at aging and cognition, family caregiving, human-computer interaction, training, functional assessment, and more. CREATE, the NIH-funded multi-site Center for Research and Education on Aging and Technology Enhancement, is only one of the projects she is involved in. It has been in existence for twenty-five years, as the necessary technology began to emerge in our everyday lives. "The center looks at aging and interactions with technology from two perspectives. One is looking at how existing and emerging technologies can support quality of life and independence for aging adults, the second is to help ensure that systems and applications are designed in so that they are usable and useful for everyday use," she explained.[28]

She and her colleagues developed a software system called PRISM (Personal Reminder Information Systems Management) that was developed to enhance social and cognitive engagement in a control group of 65-to-98-year-olds. Many of them had no prior technology experience. Study findings showed that participants who used PRISM reported less loneliness, less social isolation, and better quality of life overall. While these participants were not digital natives, I asked her if she thought today's 40-year-old would be savvier in using technology as they live to 90 or older. Czaja responded, "First of all, there is a false impression that older people are technophobic, and that couldn't be further from the truth. Technology is also dynamic. It's all going to look very different. Regardless of technology ability, younger people today are going to have to learn new things as they age. People can learn at any age; there is a lot of cognitive reserve."[29]

> **there is a false impression that older people are technophobic, and that couldn't be further from the truth**

Czaja is now working on an AI-enabled project that will allow people to ask simple queries about Medicare. With all of the complexities of understanding the system, the idea is to use technology to get accurate answers. In the study, they are also incorporating user involvement to understand the questions people might have about Medicare. Whether it is technology applications like VR, another area that she is exploring, or the multi-faceted use of AI, Czaja continues to find ways to create better lives for everyone as they age.

It's Just the Beginning

We've only just begun what will be one of the most phenomenal evolutions of medical advances that will allow all of us to live longer, healthier lives. In particular, the recent introduction of AI tools is a game changer. How these tools evolve in the coming years is likely to drive all the work at the intersection of health and technology and could lead to some truly amazing discoveries. Does that mean we will soon live in a world where reaching 100 years old is the norm? Perhaps, but it's just as likely that many of us won't see that in our lifetimes. Still, it remains a conceivable idea. The idea of the majority of the population living to 80 probably seemed unlikely in the 1930s, when life expectancy was in the low 60s, but it is now a common occurrence.[30] I don't think anyone really knows what the future of longevity looks like. For now, let's put it all in a time capsule and see what it looks like in the year 2126.

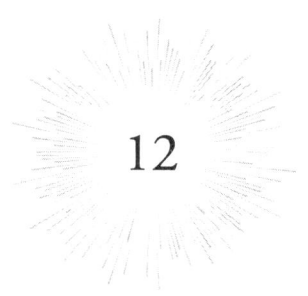

12

Improving Your Sleep to Promote Longevity

Sleep is a key factor in our quest for healthier longevity, and it has become recognized as one of the more critical aspects of our well-being. According to Dr. Els van der Helm, a Switzerland-based sleep neuroscientist, although diet and exercise have long been topics of conversations about health, sleep is now receiving equal billing.[1] In addition, Dr. Matthew Walker, a UC Berkeley neuroscientist, said in a 2018 interview, "We often think of sleep as the third pillar of good health, alongside diet and exercise. But in truth, sleep is actually the foundation on which those two other pillars will sit."[2]

Scientists, doctors, technologists, venture capitalists, for-profit companies, and nonprofits are all converging to find ways to make us all less sleep deprived. According to the CDC, one in three Americans does not get enough sleep, and globally, up to 45 percent of the population doesn't.[3] Furthermore, according to a study of 22,330 adults from thirteen countries published in *Sleep Medicine* in November 2021, one in three participants had critical insomnia symptoms and nearly 20 percent met the criteria for insomnia disorder.[4]

Although data like this has contributed to the recent increase in sleep-related conversations, the scientific study of sleep is not new.

The Science of Sleep

The modern science of sleep was developed by Dr. Nathaniel Kleitman, who studied sleep cycles and circadian rhythms at the University of Chicago in the 1920s and 30s. In 1939, he published *Sleep and Wakefulness*, which is considered the foundational work for what is the modern sleep research that we know today. He and his student Eugene Aserinsky discovered the idea of REM sleep in 1953, a critical moment in the study of sleep.[5] Other developments followed, including the discovery of melatonin by Dr. Aaron Lerner in 1958 and the classification of sleep phases by Drs. Allan Rechtschaffen and Anthony Kales in 1968.

In 1977, Dr. Peter Hauri, a clinical psychologist, developed the modern foundation of a lot of today's sleep therapies with his rules of sleep hygiene. In his book *The Sleep Disorders*, Hauri emphasized the importance of things like maintaining a regular sleep schedule, avoiding caffeine and alcohol, and having a steady amount of daily exercise.[6]

Cognitive Behavioral Therapy for Insomnia (CBT-I) was developed in the 1980s by Dr. Richard Bootzin and refined through clinical trials in the 1990s. It is now considered the gold standard for chronic insomnia and is a relevant therapy for people of all ages.

Eve Van Cauter, PhD from the University of Chicago, studies how sleep loss affects metabolism, hormones, and obesity, and has also focused some of her studies on aging. Cauter's 1999 study with several colleagues showed that just six nights of partial sleep deprivation could lead to glucose intolerance and reduced leptin levels and could "age" metabolism.[7]

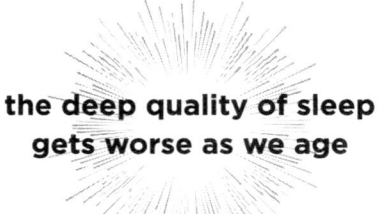

the deep quality of sleep gets worse as we age

More recently, Matthew Walker from UC Berkeley has become one of the most visible experts on the topic of sleep. His TED Talk, "Sleep Is Your Superpower," has more than fourteen million views.[8] He has been interviewed by both Joe Rogan and Dr. Andrew Huberman leading to ten million views and nearly four million views, respectively. In his TED Talk, Walker provides insight into his work on how the deep quality of sleep gets worse as we age. Some of the research in his sleep center focuses on learning, memory, and how the disruption of sleep can contribute to reduced cognition and more. Walker has also focused on aging and longevity in some of his work

While understanding why we sleep still has a lot of mystery to it, it is thanks to these researchers and others, some of whom we'll introduce later in this chapter, that we know that sleep does important work for us. The body performs a maintenance update while we sleep for the recommended seven to eight hours each night, removing toxins, repairing cellular and DNA damage, and more. It's important for brain health and ultimately for our own longevity.

Sleep Issues in Our Later Years

Even for those of us who avoided insomnia or other sleep disorder diagnoses in our youth, age-related sleep issues often arise in our later years. For example, we tend to spend less time in deep sleep and REM sleep. The body's internal clock or circadian rhythms can change, and other health issues or medications can disrupt our sleep patterns, leading to fatigue and other complications. Our sleep chronotypes also change during different phases of our lives. By the time we are in our 60s or older, we tend towards a strong morning chronotype, which means feeling sleepy earlier and waking up earlier.

Large studies have consistently shown that there are links between long-term sleep problems and early dementia, as well as early-onset Alzheimer's disease. A 2021 study in *Nature Communications* that followed thousands of people for more than twenty-five years discovered that people who had sleep problems that started in midlife and weren't addressed had a 30–40 percent higher risk of dementia later in life.[9] Furthermore, a study of 172,321 adults concluded that men who get adequate sleep live about five years longer than men who don't. For women, it's two years.[10] Better sleep equals a longer life.

Obviously, sleep is critical to our mental and physical health, so it's no wonder that the market for products that promise to help us sleep has grown to monumental proportions.

The Market for Sleep

As I set off to explore sleep as an important factor in enhancing healthy longevity, I quickly learned that there's an enormous ecosystem with so many dimensions to it that the average person can be truly overwhelmed. The amount of information, advice, opinions, services, and products that make up what is known as the global sleep industry continues to grow in exponential ways.

It has been estimated that the economic market size hit $585 billion in 2024.[11] That includes everything from mattresses to wearable devices to supplements, although the topic of sleep as part of a specific longevity agenda is hard to identify as a subset of the industry. A lot of the growth in the sleep market is being driven by new tech products, much of it fueled by AI applications. Venture capital funding for sleep tech nearly doubled between 2017 and 2021.[12] Later in this chapter, I'll cover some of the Re-Imagineer age-tech companies that are committed to finding better sleep solutions for everyone.

The global stress management market was estimated at $18.8 billion in 2023 and is projected to grow at a compound annual growth rate (CAGR) of 4–5 percent through 2031, reaching $26.7 billion.[13] This market includes mental health treatments, corporate wellness programs, and digital wellness solutions. Once again, it's hard to identify the market size of the efforts that are targeted specifically at people over 50.

There has also been a significant increase in the resources dedicated to finding ways to handle stress and calm the mind for better peace and mental relaxation, both of which have been shown to help improve stress and sleep. From ideas inspired by ancient practices to modern-day techniques, the options are boundless. And yes, there's an app for that (usually).

finding sleep solutions at a younger age has a compounding effect that will benefit people as they live longer

The supposed market size of mindfulness meditation apps varies widely depending on the source, but it's safe to say that it drives hundreds of millions of dollars in revenue, if not billions, from consumers around the world. Since longevity should be a lifelong pursuit, finding sleep solutions at a younger age has a compounding effect that will benefit people as they live longer. There was so much to sort out on the topic that I asked my friend Steve to become my research associate to help identify some meaningful insights around this topic. I also thought that what he learned might help him in solving some of his own sleep problems. (Just for the record, I'm one of those annoying people who doesn't really have any sleep issues. When my head hits the pillow, I'm out.)

While there are many sources to help solve sleeping issues, the exciting new frontier involves all forms of technology to help people address sleep, stress, and anxiety. Dr. Jenna Glover, the chief clinical officer at Headspace, explained that most of the company's engagement with customers involves stress and sleep issues.[14] Headspace offers multiple solutions, including "sleepcasts," which are audio content designed specifically to create the right conditions for healthy, restful sleep. "We have an in-depth insomnia program that takes eight weeks to complete. We also offer an eighteen-day program where people go through learning four key skills. During the program we can identify someone's sleep problems and help them with solutions," Glover said.[15]

Headspace has also begun integrating AI, introducing Ebb, an empathetic AI companion that has been trained in motivational interviewing techniques. "Ebb can help someone go through gratitude exercises, which we know is connected to healthy longevity. Ebb is also helping in mental well-being by creating social connection. Individuals come back often, relying on Ebb's understanding of them. Someone might ask Ebb to give them a sleeping solution, for example, and get a more customized response," said Glover.[16]

Sleep technology is exploding across the world, and not just with wearables like WHOOP, the Oura ring, smart watches, Google Nest, and other devices, but also with bedding, lighting, and headband wearables. According to a McKinsey report, the number of sleep-technology patents has increased by 12 percent per year over the past decade, with sleep devices alone taking the global market from $11 billion in 2019 to $32 billion by 2026.[17]

While there is still a lot of data needed to determine how these devices might help find solutions to sleeping issues, in the same report, Dr. Ingo Fietze, head of the Interdisciplinary Center of Sleep Medicine at the Charité hospital in Berlin, said, "The more we know about the sleep behavior of the population, the better we can identify intercultural and gender differences and learn about the influence of light, temperature, noise, and humidity."[18]

Resmed is a tech company that uses remote sleep-monitoring techniques and offers devices and digital health technologies to treat sleep apnea. Patients can access their personal data, use CBT applications to treat their condition, and monitor their progression. The ecosystem of digital sleep solutions also includes companies like Eight Sleep, which has created a smart mattress known as The Pod, featuring dynamic cooling and heating, detailed sleep tracking, and sleep coaching, complete with an annual digital subscription to help you better understand your sleep needs.

In both 2024 and 2025, sleep tech companies won the CES Innovation Award in Digital Health. DeRUCCI, the 2024 winner, manufactures an AI-powered smart mattress that tracks sleep and health.[19] ERA, the 2025 winner, makes the Smart Layer, a mattress topper with similar attributes.[20]

Expect to see more and more AI-generated sleep tech devices that are designed to create solutions for healthier longevity. Do they work? Only time will tell, as technologies continue to evolve, data is gathered, and final evidence-based assessments can be made. In the meantime, some consumers, such as my friend Steve Sharp, have decided to give them a shot. Since nothing else has really worked for him, he said, "Why not give it a try?"[21]

The Root of the Problem

Regardless of the sleep solution that works for you, understanding the root of the problem is what's important. In the American Psychological Association's *Stress in America* survey, 43 percent of adults reported that stress has caused them to lie awake at night.[22]

Manjit Devgun is a leading mind coach who integrates self-hypnosis, breath work, energy healing, and mindfulness techniques for her clients.[23] According to her, our breath is key to longevity. "Studies show that when you breathe deeper, longer breaths, you can increase your lung capacity, boost immunity, and add seven years to your life expectancy. You can eliminate anxiety by spending just three minutes a day breathing slowly and exhaling twice as long."[24]

In her Manjit app, she offers free guided workshop sessions on how to improve breathing for a more relaxed state. Her practice also includes ways to make behavioral changes in small increments to reduce stress and overcome obstacles that may be creating anxiety in your life.

Other solutions include Calm, Happier Meditation, and Mindfulness.com. A simple Google search can help find what most appeals to you, whether it is app-based or live gatherings.

Headspace offers multiple content collections that can help with stress and mental fitness, and when I spoke with Glover in February 2025, she emphasized the importance of community on their platform, noting that "sharing one's experience with mindfulness techniques, for example, can help others."[25]

If you're not into apps, there are also doctors who specialize in sleep disorders. To find a sleep doctor certified in sleep medicine, look for sleep centers that are accredited by the American Academy of Sleep Medicine (AASM). For sleep centers that focus on longevity, check out NYU Langone Health Brain Aging & Sleep Center and the Northwestern University Center for Circadian and Sleep Medicine.

Dr. Meeta Singh is a board-certified psychiatrist and sleep medicine specialist based in Michigan who offers a concierge approach focused on optimizing sleep as a cornerstone of longevity and performance.[26] Her exclusive clientele includes professional athletes from the NFL and NBA and high-performing C-suite executives who struggle with sleep disruption despite their disciplined lifestyles. These individuals often face unique challenges: irregular travel schedules, high-pressure decision-making environments, and the cognitive demands of elite performance, all of which can severely impact sleep quality. As a psychiatrist, she also said that focusing on sleep issues with her client is another way of getting to the root of a lot of other issues she can help with.

"As we get older, our sleep gets lighter and certain behaviors can affect our sleep. For example, naps during the day can disrupt sleep at night," she explained.[27] She's also a big proponent of using a "winding down" strategy before attempting to sleep. "Think of it as landing a plane. It loses altitude, makes the right maneuvers, loses speed, and ultimately comes in for a landing," she said, noting that it can take some people several hours to wind down enough to sleep.[28]

Better sleep through the various options we reviewed in this chapter can lead to better longevity, as can improving your mental health and reducing stress. But much of your longevity is tied into your own attitude about aging. That, too, can create a level of stress that leads to depression and unhappiness.

I interviewed Becca Levy, PhD, about her breakthrough book *Breaking the Age Code* for OprahDaily.com. Levy is professor of epidemiology at Yale School of Public Health and professor of psychology at Yale. During the interview, I had what Oprah would call an "Aha moment." Let me go right to the headline: A positive attitude about aging can lead to seven and a half more years of life![29]

much of your longevity is tied into your own attitude about aging

The *Ohio Longitudinal Study of Aging and Retirement*, done in Oxford, Ohio, tracked beliefs about aging among 433 participants between 1977 and 1995.[30] Levy took the study findings and added mortality data collected from the National Death Index to make connections between attitudes and functional health. She determined that those participants who had more positive views of aging lived seven and a half years longer on average. Positive age beliefs across all types of people conferred a better survival advantage or more longevity on average than low cholesterol, low blood pressure, low body mass index, or avoiding smoking. "In our studies, we have found that those with more positive age beliefs also performed better physically and cognitively. We also found that positive age beliefs helped people recover from injuries and periods of depression," she said.[31]

To start your own process, Levy recommends the ABC method to bolster positive age beliefs. The A stands for increasing our awareness of the ageism around us and our own age belief. The B stands for placing blame where it is due, like structural factors that we can change, and the C stands for challenging ageism in our society and culture.

Other books that can help in the quest to combat internal age-ism and reduce anxiety (and probably make you sleep better) include *Mindfulness for Beginners: Reclaiming the Present Moment—And Your Life* by Jon Kabat-Zinn, and Swedish writer Magareta Magnusson's *The Swedish Art of Aging Exuberantly: Life Wisdom from Someone Who Will (Probably) Die Befor You.*

What we know is that our longevity is deeply tied to better sleep, less stress, and a consistently healthy mental state. Fortunately, there are a number of science-based sleep hacks you can use to improve your sleep.

Some Simple Sleep Hacks

Since it was first proposed in 1977 by Dr. Peter Hauri, the concept of sleep hygiene has continued to evolve and adapt to contemporary life to include the following checklist of sleep and longevity hacks. This is not an exhaustive list, but I put these together by studying recommendations from multiple sources:

- Keep a regular sleep schedule. Go to bed and wake up at the same time every day. It helps with your circadian rhythm, especially as it changes as you age.
- Alcohol, caffeine, nicotine, and heavy meals can impact your sleep. Doctors and organizations like the Cleveland Clinic recommend no alcohol three to four hours before you go to sleep. When we age, we often have fragmented sleep, and these stimulants can reduce sleep quality.
- Keep your room quiet, cool, and dark. (I am known to turn on the air conditioner in winter as a way to cool down the room.) The kind of bed you sleep on is important too.
- Exercise during the day can promote better sleep. Any kind of movement is important, not just for sleep but for your overall health. My exercise regimen tends to be later in the day, so my thesis is that this helps me sleep better at night.
- Try to reduce stress by winding down before you go to sleep. Using meditation apps, sitting in a still position, and concen-

trating on your breathing can help. Some people stretch or do yoga to move into their preparation for bedtime.

- Try to avoid using technology in bed (I'm really bad at this one). My friend Carolyn puts all of her devices, including her phone, in another room before she goes to sleep! I'm in awe.
- As people age, it's even more important to be exposed to both morning and dusk light to maintain circadian rhythms. It helps in your sleep cycle.

As part of this discussion of solutions designed to promote better sleep, it's worth noting that many sleep experts do not believe that sleeping pills provide the important natural sleep. Instead, sleeping pills have the potential to damage our health and increase the risk of life-threatening diseases. As people age, sleeping pills can also contribute to dizziness (leading to falls), impact cognitive issues, and create an addiction. With a doctor's advice, better solutions might include natural supplements like melatonin, magnesium (which can help calm the nervous system), or even chamomile tea to create a state of relaxation.

The Future of Sleep

The big opportunity for the future is researching the connections between all of these ideas for longevity. While we know that aging impacts certain aspects of sleep, wouldn't finding ways to reduce those impacts be the next big revolution in sleep science? What if there are breakthroughs that challenge the prevailing knowledge about aging and sleep? Whether it is from a neuroscientist, a venture capitalist funding new techniques, or an age tech company, it doesn't matter where a solution comes from. The next generation of innovators will become known as the sleep Re-Imagineers for a longevity nation.

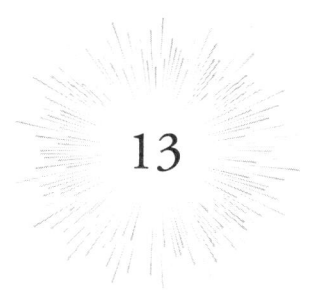

13

Diet and Exercise:
The Longevity Lifestyle

When I first met Dr. Peter Attia, he was about to be interviewed by Oprah for her Oprah Daily platform about his book *Outlive: The Science and Art of Longevity*. The book had just come out and would eventually become a worldwide bestseller. In the green room before he took the stage at Hearst Tower in New York, I told him that I had just finished reading the book and that the message resonated with me, especially that we should all live our lives to set the groundwork for our "Centenarian Decathlon."[1] I would soon be leaving for the Tenzing Hillary Everest Marathon, so I shared some examples of how I had trained, along with my diet and healthy habits that prepared me for the adventure.

If you are interested in longevity, you already know that how often and what kind of exercise you do and what you eat each day are cornerstones for your healthy life. Add to that sleep, stress reduction, community, and purpose, and you have the road map for extending your own personal longevity journey.

Why this is so important is that there are multiple studies and supporting research that have established that only 25 percent of your longevity is determined by genetics, with the remaining due to lifestyle, environment, and other factors.[2] So, if your parents lived well into their 90s, you might have a head start, but it's unlikely to be enough to carry you into your 90s or beyond if you don't pay attention to the 75 percent that you can control. To that end, let's take a closer look at the role of exercise and diet in longevity.

Exercising for Longevity

Ask any expert and you'll learn that movement is one of the most critical elements of healthy aging, or as Weill Cornell Doctor Mark Lachs says, "motion is lotion."

While I'm a marathon runner who also lifts weights, cycles, and skis, that's the program that works for me, and I know I have to maintain my regimen throughout my life. It doesn't mean that you must train for a marathon, but it does mean that during the week you should have some type of program that includes aerobics, flexibility, mobility, and weight training for strength.

Forget the debate about whether ten thousand steps is the right or wrong metric—just get out there and do something, even if it's what some people call "exercise snacks." That means take the stairs, do squats while you're on a call, stand on one foot for as long as you can while you're cooking, stretch out on the floor, or do crunches while you're watching your favorite television series. Even doing it in ten-minute increments several times a day is meaningful.

According to Dr. Michael Fredericson, movement and exercise is the number one focus for healthy longevity, and he advocates that it is never too late to start.[3] A professor and director of Physical Medicine and Rehabilitation in the Department of Orthopaedic Surgery at Stanford University, he works with people of all ages.

"The goal should be 150 minutes a week of moderate aerobic exercise or 75 minutes of vigorous exercise, including two days of resistance training for at least 30 minutes. We should do this from the age of 18 until we die. For people over 65, add in balance exercises. Tai chi, yoga and Pilates are all great ways to build strength and balance," he said.[4]

While his suggestions are a great starting point, at 66, his own routine includes tai chi and karate (he is an eighth-degree blackbelt), which he says is great conditioning for strength, flexibility, and having to learn complex movements (which is good for brain health). He also swims, bikes, and lifts weights a couple of times a week. Fredericson is also excited about the developments in platelet-rich plasma injections for healing sports or other injuries. These will become precision-based approaches for the individual, extending overall health and the ability to continue to exercise.

All around us there are inspirational Re-Imagineers who started a fitness regimen in the second halves of their lives. For example, Joan MacDonald started her workouts at 71, after watching her mother struggle with the ability to move.[5] Supported by her daughter, who is in the fitness business, she set off on her own journey to live a better life or, as she puts it, "You can't turn back the clock, but you can wind it up again."[6] MacDonald started with a "transformation group" of other women, doing yoga once a week and four days of weight training for strength. Within a year, she lost seventy pounds and improved her overall health metrics enough to allow her to go off several medications. She became such an inspiration that she now has two million followers on Instagram with the tagline, "Showing you that it's never too late to become your strongest self."

> **You can't turn back the clock, but you can wind it up again**

"In the beginning, a lot of my followers were in their 30s, and they told me they would show their parents or aunts or uncles what I was doing, to get them involved in an exercise regimen," she said.[7] Now 80 years old, MacDonald continues to inspire with her Train with Joan app. She also landed a cover story on *Women's Health* magazine to show women of all ages what is possible.

Tim Minnick, another Re-Imagineer who started working out later in life, was in his 60s when he lost his wife to breast cancer.[8] To deal with his grief, along with his own health and weight issues, he began going to a local gym. Not only did it lead to a complete transformation, but it also gave him a new purpose in life. He decided to become a fitness trainer in his 70s and began applying for jobs in his hometown of Austin, Texas. "We often let society influence our thoughts about aging. We limit ourselves and say things like 'I can't do that because of my age.' I believe in just the opposite," he said.[9]

Not only did he land a job, but at 82, he is now recognized by the *Guinness Book of World Records* as the world's oldest fitness trainer. He has become a role model for reinvention, lifelong fitness, and health span.

One of the biggest trends in longevity nations is the rise of longevity gyms, which take a holistic view of exercise and lifestyle. Some examples include Love.Life in El Segundo, California; MIORA in Minneapolis, Minnesota; and Optimize by Equinox, first launched in New York City and Highland Park, Texas. All of them integrate workouts with nutrition, comprehensive evaluations of sleep patterns, VO2 max tests, bloodwork, and AI-generated wellness plans that are created on an individualized basis. With the rise of GLP-1 usage, there are even gyms that offer fitness plans focused on users of the drug. Planet Fitness and Xponential are only two examples of fitness chains that are moving into this space.

While these are next-gen versions of the exercise sector, it is still the simple act of moving that will keep you healthier longer. Call it old-school, but a long walk on the beach or cycling in your local park is still a key practice to building your own longevity plan.

Renee J. Rogers, PhD, FACSM, is a senior scientist at the University of Kansas Medical Center. An expert in bio-behavioral healthy lifestyles, some of her research focuses on sedentary individuals and how exercise can change them as they age.[10] When I spoke with her in May 2025, she said, "We recruit people who are inactive and have never done anything. It allows us to see the benefits and impact that movement can have on someone who is starting a healthy lifestyle program."[11]

In her work, she considers how body composition and muscle mass change as we age, along with what works for the individual for the moment that they are in now. That might mean not starting someone right into an exercise program. "We encourage people over 50 who have never exercised to start by taking movement breaks. There's a lot of research that shows that even ten minutes of movement can be beneficial. As more time is added, it leads to better outcomes."[12]

As we live longer, sarcopenia becomes more of a critical issue. Sarcopenia is loss of muscle mass, which can impact strength and function. It's amplified by a lack of movement/exercise in combination with aging.

Dr. Gabrielle Lyon created Muscle-Centric Medicine to strengthen muscle for people of all ages. She is a clinical practitioner and the author of *Forever Strong: A New, Science-Based Strategy for Aging Well*.[13] She is also an educator and science communicator and has a podcast that is dedicated to exploring the science of muscles, nutrition, and longevity. When I spoke to her in May 2025, Lyon said, "Diseases begin in the skeletal muscle, the largest organ system in the body. Muscle span—the length of time that you live with a healthy and robust skeletal system—is critical to health span and a quality lifespan."[14] Lyon says that building muscle as we age, in combination with a diet that supports muscles, is key to longevity. That includes high-quality proteins. The aging phenomenon happens in muscles but can be overcome with a combination of training and whole foods high in quality proteins, according to her.

building muscle as we age, in combination with a diet that supports muscles, is key to longevity

Lyon is also concerned about rising use of GLP-1 drugs, as one of the side effects is muscle loss. The long-term effects of these drugs, especially on older people, is not yet known. According to Lyons, "It may lead to another type of epidemic of frailty and osteoporosis. There will have to be other medications, some kind of anabolic agent that will balance it out. They will help to preserve and protect muscle for those who use GLP-1 drugs."[15]

We will discuss GLP-1 drugs more later in this chapter. Regardless of one's medications, exercise remains an important component of longevity. But, as Lyon notes, exercise alone is not enough; your diet also plays a critical role in longevity. Furthermore, there's an important interrelationship between exercise and eating critical elements when it comes to building your own longevity lifestyle.

Eating for Longevity

How we should eat, when we should eat, and what we should eat as we age is a maze of information that can confuse anyone. One study says one thing and another study contradicts it. There are lots of experts with lots of views on what is best for a healthier life.

The book *Outlive* says it best: "We actually don't know that much about how what we eat affects our health."[16] It advocates for "Nutritional Biochemistry," an approach that I prefer and practice. You can read more about it in that book.

The Mediterranean diet, rich in vegetables, fruits, legumes, and olive oil, is often viewed as one of the best for longevity. Another is the Blue Zones diet, which is mostly plant based, and the MIND diet (Mediterranean-DASH diet intervention for neurodegenerative delay) supports brain health and reduces the risk of cognitive decline and Alzheimer's.

Separately, a recent major trend extolls the virtues of what are known as functional foods and beverages, which contain ingredients specifically targeted at promoting longevity and addressing age-related concerns. Many functional foods, such as yogurts, kefir, miso, and kombucha tea, contain probiotics, prebiotics, and other compounds that positively influence the gut microbiome. Others may contain ashwagandha, quercetin, L-theanine, and curcumin, which are all believed to support various aspects of healthy aging.

Choline, an essential nutrient, is also gaining attention in the study of food and longevity as it promotes brain health, liver function, and cellular integrity. One study in the *American Journal of Clinical Nutrition* (2011) found that people with higher choline intake performed better on memory tests, as choline produces acetylcholine, an important neurotransmitter also involved in muscle movement and regulating heartbeat.[17] Everyday foods that are high in choline include eggs, soybeans, and Atlantic cod.

To learn more about the connection between diet and longevity, in September 2024 I spoke with Valter Longo, a biogerontologist (someone who studies the biology of aging). Longo is a professor of gerontology and biological sciences and director of the Longevity Institute at USC and the Program on Longevity and Cancer in Milan, Italy, as well as the cofounder of a Biology of Aging PhD program at USC. He is also the author of *The Longevity Diet*, an international bestseller that proposes an everyday diet based on five pillars of longevity, combined with a scientifically engineered plant-based fasting-mimicking diet three or four times a year to extend healthy lifespan.[18]

His ongoing research and clinical trials have led to a unique approach on how nutritional interventions can promote cellular repair and reduce disease risk. In his book, he promotes a concept called programmed longevity: a biological strategy that protects and regenerates cells. When you program your health through his approach, your body's systems will trigger protection, repair, and replacement mechanisms to maintain your vigor and functionality. Some of the key elements of the longevity diet include following a pescetarian diet that is close to 100 percent plant and fish based; consuming low but sufficient proteins, such as those in legumes and nuts; and maximizing good fats and complex carbs like salmon and olive oil. "Our longevity diet has components of the Mediterranean, Okinawa, and Loma Linda diets, but is specifically designed for minimizing disease and maximizing a healthy lifespan," he told me when we spoke in September.[19]

Longo also advocates for time-restricted eating and periodic, prolonged fasting to optimize healthy longevity. "We created a five-day meal program called Prolon, a concept that is designed to mimic the effects of a water-only fast while still providing essential nutrients," he explained.[20] Longo developed the Prolon program to help reboot metabolism, and he donates 100 percent of his consulting fees for it to the Create Cures Foundation.

The world of nutrition and its impact on longevity is expected to continue to expand due to a growing emphasis on preventive health measures that can be augmented by good eating. Eric Williamson is at the center of this trend as the director of nutrition for Canyon Ranch and a leader in the LONGEVITY8™ program, a four-day retreat that focuses on eight key pillars of well-being and health.[21] Williamson's education, which includes two undergraduate degrees in kinesiology and nutrition and dietetics and an MSc and PhD in exercise nutrition and metabolism, along with multiple certifications in nutrition and fitness, informs his approach to establishing a link between nutrition and longevity. "My focus is on the role of individual nutrients, food groups, and overall diet in longevity and to identify key foods that will give each specific person the greatest return on investment for their long-term health," Williamson explained.[22]

This means focusing on a diet filled with more whole foods and less processed food and refined sugar. According to Williamson, achieving an optimal nutrient-dense diet improves life length because it contributes to other outcomes associated with health, such as aerobic fitness, high muscle mass, and a lean body fat percentage. "Beans are more related to a longer lifespan than any other food group. They are nutrient dense with fiber and protein and high in antioxidants, phyto-nutrients, and vitamins and minerals. All beans are good, and they are accessible and affordable," he said.[23]

While all our bodies have different needs, Williamson believes that finding an approach that is personalized to an individual's body, life-style, and schedule is in our future. MyFitnessPal and RxFood are two examples of apps that already use AI-powered tools to monitor nutrient intake and make recommendations. The use of a continuous glucose monitor for longevity enthusiasts is another way to identify specific foods that allow a person to better control their glucose level. In the near future, Williamson believes we'll have smart glasses with integrated AI that will track how much you eat throughout the day and estimate your nutrient intake with surprising accuracy. With the help of AI and our own diagnostic data and tools, we'll all be able to have personalized food and diet plans for our own biology.

As part of my discussion with Williamson, one of the things I wanted to explore is the role of alcohol as we age. There are conflicting studies and differing points of view that are all supported with different research. When I asked Williamson about this, he responded:

> In my longevity presentations, I recommend that people quan-tify everything, especially in nutrition. Many populations that drink alcohol are some of the longest-living populations. It is a part of their communal experience and culture, and we know that the number one predictor of a longer life is our relation-ships. Many factors influence how alcohol affects a person's health. If you have no diseases, eat nutritiously, exercise regu-larly, and maintain strong social relationships, your risk from

moderate alcohol intake will look very different compared to someone who doesn't share those habits. [24]

In *Outlive*, it is noted that the lifestyle around moderate drinking can also help relieve stress. It encourages people to be mindful about it, limiting alcohol to fewer than seven servings per week, and ideally no more than two on any given day.[25]

Personally, I enjoy wine and an occasional margarita. There are also foods that are not on the "longevity preferred list" that I still want to eat, including a great Tex-Mex meal and crispy french fries. I'm willing to take the risk, as the joy of good food and wine is important to me, as it is to many of my family and friends as we gather as a community to share our lives. Ultimately, it is the individual's responsibility to embrace an exercise regimen and gain an understanding of the foods we should eat, the alcohol we consume, and the risks associated with those decisions.

The Rise of GLP-1 Drugs

At the intersection of weight, diet, exercise, and emerging longevity benefits is the revolution of GLP-1 drugs, which are impacting so many lives in a positive way. Whether it is Wegovy, Ozempic, Zepbound, or a handful of other medications, it's just the beginning of what will be a profound change in how we treat obesity and related chronic diseases. As medication costs come down, new affordable pill forms are introduced, more alternatives are developed, and commercial insurance plans and Medicare ultimately cover the cost for more patients, it will democratize obesity treatment for millions, helping them live longer, healthier lives.

Dr. Katherine H. Saunders is a physician innovator and internationally recognized expert in obesity medicine. She is also cofounder of FlyteHealth, a precision cardiometabolic care solution spanning obesity, diabetes, hypertension, and related comorbidities, using data and AI to enable cost-effective, scalable, and self-sustaining treatment models nationwide. She described the need for medical intervention in obesity treatment: "If you take a look at the dietary interventions, average weight loss is only 3–5 percent, and more than half of the weight is regained within two years. By five years, more than 80 percent is regained. Most people with obesity require medical intervention to lose a clinically significant amount of weight and maintain that weight loss long-term."[26]

GLP-1s have completely changed the game as interventions that not only help reduce weight but can also impact longevity. Since obesity is a major risk factor for diabetes, strokes, heart attacks, and accelerated aging, these drugs also improve or resolve weight-related complications and decrease the risk of developing new weight-related chronic issues, according to Saunders. She notes that obesity is a complex, heterogenous, chronic disease, which means that every individual should be evaluated and treated with personalized protocols that include a range of medications, varying dosages, and long-term support.

> **Most people with obesity require medical intervention to lose a clinically significant amount of weight and maintain that weight loss long-term**

"Aside from treating obesity, GLP-1 recepter agonists confer additional benefits such as improving sleep apnea, reducing cardiovascular risk, and even controlling a variety of addictions. Most of my patients on GLP-1 drink less alcohol, and I even have a patient whose gambling addiction has been in check since he started Zepbound. There is a growing body of evidence that GLP-1s can be effective on the addiction front," she said.[27]

However, Saunders emphasizes that lifestyle interventions are still critical for health and longevity, noting, "Stopping smoking is the number one best thing you can do. It's also important to develop healthy and sustainable eating habits and engage in plenty of physical activity. These behaviors cannot be replaced by a shot or a pill."[28]

Find the Best Solution for You

Along with sleep, exercise and a healthy diet are important keys to longevity. Fortunately, there are countless studies, experts, and even apps that can help you. Focus on finding exercise and eating approaches that intersect with the best research, and use personalization and AI applications to enhance your experience. However, it is recommenced that you do this with the help of your physician, a nutritionist, and a professional trainer. You might even consider seeking out a sleep doctor. All of these professionals are there to help you create your individual journey. It is possible for everyone in a longevity nation to live their best life to 100 or older. Find your path, follow your favorite advisors, and keep it evidence based. Let's go raise some health together!

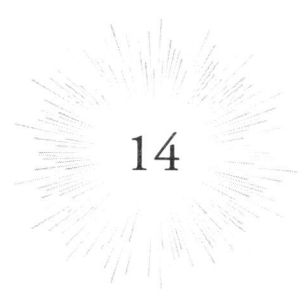

14

Skin Longevity:
A New Frontier of Discovery

I t's well established that there is a correlation between healthy skin and longevity. The care of our skin, the largest organ in our body, is interconnected with our overall health. Ask any doctor and you will learn that those who have good skin health are usually the healthiest people, and healthy skin is determined by your overall health.

For this chapter, I decided to focus on facial skin, as it has so many multi-dimensional aspects to explore, especially as we live longer. Our faces are usually how we are first perceived by others as we go through the aging process, and they are also how we perceive ourselves. It's a combination of physical, emotional, and psychological factors that conjure up all kinds of thoughts when we look in the mirror.

If you want to start an interesting conversation at a dinner party, ask your tablemates if they believe in any kind of treatments, noninvasive or invasive, for the face and why? What I've learned is that many people over 50 who can afford it have all tried something, whether it was a chemical peel, Botox, laser treatments, injectables, or other treatments. When I've asked why, the answers have been some version of to improve self-esteem, to get rid of spots or sun damage, to feel refreshed, to look younger, or to deal with some type of inherited condition like dark circles under the eyes.

Given their obvious popularity, I was curious to learn what might be happening with new treatments and technologies to keep our faces looking healthier longer. You'll note that I didn't say youthful, which is certainly one of the key motivators for many people, but rather healthy. What should a 60-, 70-, 80-, or 90-year-old face look like as a healthy reflection of that individual? And what should we do about it?

The True Goal: Healthy Skin

Martha McCully is the founding beauty director of *Allure*, the leading magazine brand in the category, and is now a beauty wellness writer and consultant. In her 60s, she has seen it all, covered it all, and tried a lot of products and treatments over the years. She has also been at the forefront of the pro-aging, healthy aging, and beautiful aging movement, a leader in rejecting the line "anti-aging."

"It seems the intensity of wrinkle-scrutiny happens in our 50s, kind of as a last gasp, when we are at the peak of that balance of vanity and wisdom, before we are too busy to care less," she said.[1] She adds that, while she has her own regimen, "none of it makes me feel as good as just being in my present life, happy in my own skin, something that paradoxically comes with age."[2]

Valerie Monroe spent sixteen years as the beauty director at *O, the Oprah Magazine* and now writes a newsletter entitled *How Not to F*ck Up Your Face: Philosophical and Practical Advice for Anyone Who's Ever Looked into a Mirror* (found at valeriemonroe.substack.com). She is in her 70s and suggests to her readers that they should learn to see their face with less objectification.[3] "Mirror meditation is a great way to see ourselves in new ways with increasing self-acceptance. I follow Tara Well, a psychologist who wrote *Mirror Meditation: The Power of Neuroscience and Self-Reflection to Overcome Self-Criticism, Gain Confidence, and See Yourself with Compassion*," she said.[4] Monroe's healthy skin regimen advice is to use a good moisturizer, a Retin-A product, an alpha hydroxy acid or beta hydroxy acid once a week, and sunscreen. She uses a combined moisturizer and sunscreen.

Everyone I interviewed gave this advice: Whatever your pathway or choice of products or treatments, find out what works best for you as an individual. Test and learn. There are hundreds, if not thousands, of product options already on the market that are sold in drugstores and department stores, online, and at med spas and doctors' offices. And soon, there will be specific precision treatments created just for you based on your personal phenotype, which includes your wrinkle formation, texture, and pigmentation; your genotype, or genetic makeup; and the totality of your environmental exposures, which is known as skin exposome. Imagine a day when you will have your own personalized formulas

Whatever your pathway or choice of products or treatments, find out what works best for you as an individual

to maintain your healthy skin as you age, combining genetics, DNA-based skin tests, biomarker tracking, nanocosmeceuticals, and more, all enhanced with AI capabilities.

Some of the leading researchers into skin longevity initiatives include the Korea Institute of Science and Technology in Seoul, the RIKEN Center for Biosystems Dynamics Research Institute in Japan, and the Max Planck Institute for Biology of Ageing in Germany. In addition, universities from Stanford to Harvard to the Universities of Zurich and São Paulo also conduct research on the topic, as do major beauty companies like Estée Lauder, L'Oréal, Amorepacific, and Procter & Gamble.

Dr. Anne Chang and Dr. Zakia Rahman are both professors of dermatology at Stanford University School of Medicine and researchers with active clinical practices focused on skin longevity. Their research topics include retinoids, which make facial skin look healthier, laser-assisted delivery of the topical drug rapamycin for longevity, and multi-omics that reveal how cellular metabolism and inflammation interact during aging or disease.[5]

Chang also investigates the human genetics of healthy skin. In an interview on the Stanford campus, she told me that 50 percent of the way our skin looks is genetic and that skin aging genes are not the same as the genes that help determine our lifespan.[6] Her clinical research in skin aging and longevity includes understanding gene changes that predispose some people to younger-looking skin. At a Stanford Medicine Alumni day in 2023, she presented "The Genetics of Healthy Skin Aging," a talk that can be accessed on YouTube. In the video, she presents findings that might lead to solutions to reverse skin aging, using broadband light that alters some skin genes she calls "rejuvenation genes."[7]

Separately, Chang advocates for older people to continue to have skin checks. "Only 20 percent of older people see dermatologists. The encouraging news is that there are now free apps that let people take a photo and download . . . information on concerning skin conditions," she said.[8] SkinVision and Aysa from VisualDX are two examples of this type of app. However, they should only be used for gathering information to bring to the doctor's office, not to diagnose or treat a skin condition. Despite the wonders of AI, accurate diagnosis and treatment still require the experience and specialized knowledge of a licensed dermatologist.

To help make it possible for everyone to access a dermatologist, free and low-cost clinics have been started in many cities. The Anne Kastor Brooklyn Free Clinic in New York and the Health and Hope Clinic in Pensacola, Florida, are just two examples. A Google search in your area will help you identify places you can go for dermatological help.

When I asked Rahman what someone over 50 or 60 should be thinking about with regard to healthier skin, she had three great tips:

First, having a sense of agency. There is no expiration date on skin, meaning it's never too late to repair your skin, regardless of your age. Use over-the-counter treatments for sun protection and a topical regimen that includes some type of retinoid product. Also, see a dermatologist for checkups. Second, eat healthy. We know that carotenoids in foods are beneficial for skin and convert to Vitamin A. If you eat things that are healthy, studies show you look healthier and more attractive. [Some foods with high carotenoids include carrots, butternut squash, apricots, and cantaloupe.] Third, take some cues from younger people, who are very cognizant of their skin health. Their regimens are impressive. Even a three-step regimen can do wonders for improving the functioning of skin. Skin that looks better actually functions better, too, so it's a win-win scenario.[9]

The ultimate goal is to find better solutions for healthier skin, particularly as we age. The earlier someone starts, the more it creates a compounding effect for when they are older.

Additionally, since most people over 50 grew up in a time when sunscreen was not viewed as a necessity (remember baby oil and reflectors as a way to get a tan?), regular check-ups should be a part of every health routine. As a two-time skin cancer survivor, I'm always harping on people to get their skin checked and to do any kind of treatment that will help them keep their skin healthy. It's my public service message in this chapter to get on this right away, especially since I've had several friends who ignored suspicious growths on their skin and died from skin cancer.

My own daily regimen is a great cleansing soap, some skin repair products, and lots of sunscreen. More men need to focus on taking care of their skin, something that many of us weren't taught but need to learn, especially as we age.

Cutting-Edge Skincare Technology

When the subject of plastic surgery comes up, inevitably the conversation turns to who has gotten the best or worst plastic surgery. I'm always amazed at how this topic elicits such vociferous opinions and judgments from both men and women. Some of the comments, especially about celebrities over 50, are downright vicious. Ultimately, shouldn't we all just let people do what they think is best for them and what makes them feel better? It's all about freedom of expression, regardless of what it does to their expression!

The US cosmetic surgery market was $16.73 billion in 2023 and is projected to grow at a CAGR of 4.3 percent.[10] As populations age, more people may choose to go this route. The most popular surgical procedures in the United States are liposuction, breast augmentation, and tummy tucks, according to the American Society of Plastic Surgeons, followed by breast lifts and eyelid surgery.[11]

Dr. Haideh Hirmand, MD, FACS, is a Harvard-trained physician who trained in plastic surgery, with specialty training in oculoplastic and craniofacial surgeries.[12] She has had a private practice in New York since 2000 and is known for her pioneering work with both the eyes and the face, as well as aesthetic technologies. While she performs both surgical and nonsurgical procedures, her keen interest is in tissue regeneration and disruptive technologies, which now comprise at least 50 percent of her practice. As she told me during a discussion in May 2025, "Working with an individual's autologous fat, for example, works differently than surgery because it actually regenerates and repairs tissue in the face."[13] Some of the other treatments she offers incorporate PRP, or platelet-rich plasma, which stimulates collagen and elastin production, is anti-inflammatory, and is used for facial rejuvenation to improve skin texture and fine wrinkles.

According to Hirmand, cutting-edge treatments include the creation of nanofat taken from a patient's own adipose tissue and microneedled into the skin to stimulate regeneration and collagen production and improve pigmentation and tone. Exosomes are another nanoparticle treatment that can reduce wrinkles and improve tone, Hirmand explained:

> Exosomes are the new kid on the block for regeneration. They are bilayered vesicles and cells that mediate cellular communication. Exosomes can be procured from many sources including plant, animal, or human resources. One's own adipose tissue is a rich source of autologous exosomes, for example. We use them for aesthetic purposes after a procedure like laser resurfacing to hasten recovery and decrease redness.[14]

While the research is still emerging, the indication is that exosomes will restore healthier skin at a cellular level and promote skin longevity. Companies that offer exosome products include BENEV, Exocel Bio, and Kimera Labs. Countries like South Korea and Japan already use exosomes in regenerative medical practices.

Always on the lookout for new treatments that may be breakthroughs, Hirmand is also working on a clinical study through an institutional review board in collaboration with Acorn Biolabs, a Canadian company. According to her, "Acorn has figured out how to harvest stem cells that are associated with hair follicles, which contain rich cell types that include keratinocytes, fibroblasts, and mesenchymal stem cells, representing the only method so far to harvest stem cells non-invasively. They cryopreserve the cells and can then activate and culture the cells at a later time, to develop a personalized serum, a secretome, from the individual's own preserved cell," she said.[15] While there are no clinical studies completed just yet as to the efficacy in improving skin parameters, it's another approach being tested that may be helpful for healthier skin.

Hirmand is also excited about how big data and AI platforms will help determine how an individual is destined to show signs of aging as they live longer, and how she can intercept it at any point with new kinds of treatments. "Moving forward, we'll see precision longevity aesthetics that will include epigenetic, genomic, and phenotype components for an individual's treatment," she explained.[16]

For her, healthy facial skin regardless of age is all about decreasing inflammation and thickening the dermis, which is the middle layer of skin just below the epidermis. She is also focused on helping patients over 60 achieve healthier skin that reflects how they feel, saying, "For my patients over 60, the majority of them tell me that they are okay with their age. They want to look in the mirror and see a reflection of what's inside them, not some other version. There's nothing more ridiculous than trying to make a 60-year-old look 30."[17]

Dr. Steve Dayan is another skin-focused Re-Imagineer who is searching for new ways to help his patients achieve healthier skin. A Chicago-based facial plastic surgeon and author of six books, including the *New York Times* bestseller *Subliminally Exposed*, Dayan also taught a course at DePaul University called the Science of Beauty and has a long list of accolades and accomplishments in his field. Dayan is also excited about the trends in skin rejuvenation and bioregenerative products, such as Sculptra and Radiesse, both of which stimulate collagen production.[18] While there have been multiple clinical trials, he notes definitive outcomes on all the emerging biostimulators are still forthcoming. "We know that skin looks great, but we are still working on how it exactly leads to better, healthier skin," he explained when we spoke in February 2025.[19]

They want to look in the mirror and see a reflection of what's inside them

Like others in the field, Dayan is also tracking exosomes, polynucleotides, and different types of nutraceuticals that are products derived from food sources as ways to improve healthy skin elasticity, hydration, and inflammation reduction over time. One specific area he is interested in is how Ozempic and other GLP-1s are causing fat loss and rapid facial aging. "We are interested in exploring the dermal white adipose tissue, a thin layer of fat that's just under the superficial layer of skin. Within that layer are rich, nutrient cells that may get turned off by GLP-1s," he explained.[20] To address this issue, Dayan and other researchers are investigating ways to improve fillers and promote growth factors and pro-insulin cytokines in the affected area.

Dayan is also interested in the confluence of physical appearance, emotional well-being, and social perception, which has led him to launch a skincare concept that uses what he calls "Moodceuticals." They are a range of topicals designed to promote better skin health while simultaneously improving mood, attractiveness, and sexual satisfaction. The first of these, XOMD, has undergone a rigorous trial process that yielded astonishing data. According to Dayan, "By incorporating a jasmine derivative mimicking the benefits of oxytocin, which is known as a love hormone, we can improve not only skin appearance, but also levels of self-confidence."[21]

The advances in skincare technology in recent years have been profound, a trend that is expected to continue.

Longevity Skincare Products

Even though many people may not be able to afford or have access to cutting-edge products and technologies, there are companies that have invested hundreds of millions of dollars in skin science to bring more affordable products to people who want to improve their skin. The Estée Lauder Companies and L'Oréal Groupe are just two examples.

Estée Lauder has been at the forefront of skin longevity, according to Jennifer Palmer, senior vice president of Global Skincare Category and Brand Scientific Authority Strategy. "We started longevity skin science research more than fifteen years ago through inspiration from our partnerships with longevity researchers at MIT and Harvard medical school. In their work on sirtuins, we were interested in how that relates to skin and how your skin can look its best at any age," she explained.[22]

Sirtuins are proteins present in all human cells. They are involved in metabolism and control of inflammation, which play key roles in aging.[23] "Sirtuins were found to be highly activated in centenarians. They are even nicknamed the longevity protein," Palmer said. "We set out to identify sirtuin activators that activate that longevity protein in the skin."[24]

With forty-four patents worldwide and twenty-five publications and conferences on the role of sirtuins in skin, Estée Lauder has advanced its understanding of the biology of skin aging, Palmer says.[25] At the Estée Lauder Research & Development labs, researchers show how breakthrough science can slow down and even reverse skin aging on a cellular level. For example, Estée Lauder has proven that a sitruin-activating ingredient can extend the cell's active lifespan by 35 percent. Data from other research shows this technology is able to reverse key cellular measurements, such as cell shape, by twenty-three years. (Meaning a 45-year-old's skin cells can regain the shape of a 22-year-old's cells again!)

Estée Lauder also has several studies in the works with Stanford University's Program on Aesthetics & Culture to help build the data-driven foundation from which to shape the future of aesthetics and extend skin health span. One study is exploring the impact of self-perception as we age. On their Skin Longevity Institute website, Estée Lauder continues to educate consumers on all aspects of longevity, as well as build out the concept in key retail and travel destinations around the world.

L'Oréal Groupe, the Paris-based global beauty company, also has a longevity strategy for skin. Vania Lacascade, who earned a PhD in pharmacy as well as an MBA, is the former chief innovation officer at L'Oréal.[26] In this role, she developed strategic innovation road maps for all L'Oréal divisions. She recently became the new Lancôme global brand president. When we spoke about recent innovations in longevity skin-care at L'Oréal in April 2025, she told me how beauty connects to health:

Beauty is integral to overall health, playing a pivotal role in that intersection, particularly now that we better understand the various hallmarks of aging that are specific to skin. We are now going beyond the skin's surface to target the root causes of biological aging. Our multi-faceted approach extends skin cellular health span in unprecedented ways. We call this L'Oréal Longevity Integrative Sciences."[27]

After fifteen years of research and forty-three publications, L'Oréal has created the "Wheel of Longevity for Beauty," which decodes skin biological aging at the cellular, molecular, and tissular levels. This model allows them to explore the secrets of the nine interconnected hallmarks of aging using a proprietary Longevity AI Cloud™ to better understand the role of each and identify integrative beauty solutions and protocols. "For example, mitochondria are essential for skin health, acting as the 'powerhouses' within skin cells. Their activity, responsible for generating 90 percent of cellular energy, declines with age. When mitochondrial activity decreases, reactivation is key to producing optimal energy levels for youthful-looking skin," she explained.[28]

Finding integrative solutions for each personalized skin biological journey is what she and the four thousand L'Oréal Research and Innovation scientists focus on. This has led to the launch of the Lancôme Absolue Longevity Soft Cream, inspired by the groundbreaking skin booster technology of PDRN (polydeoxyribonucleotide), a DNA-derived compound proven effective in tissue repair and anti-inflammatory applications that is widely used in regenerative medicine and aesthetic dermatology.

Personalized skin diagnostics are also key at L'Oréal. L'Oréal unveiled Cell BioPrint at the 2025 CES show. It's a portable "lab-on-a-chip" biological diagnosis device, enabling consumers to understand their aging trajectory and identify skincare solutions to potentially reverse their skin's biological age. "This quick, five-minute skin diagnosis uses advanced proteomics to understand your individual aging process and reveal your skin needs," Lacascade said.[29] Developed in partnership with the South Korean company, NanoEntek, Cell Bio-Print will be a part of a pilot program with a L'Oréal brand in 2026, with the goal of a global rollout.

Other partnerships include strong collaborations with Timeline, a Swiss longevity biotech company specializing in mitochondria, along with TruDiagnostic, an epigenetic testing company, and the biotech company SENISCA, which develops innovations targeting senescence.

According to Lacascade, L'Oréal is focused on a new era for beauty where skin biological age is the new truth. This is just the beginning of the new era of the beauty longevity story.

Looking to the Future of Skin Longevity

The Re-Imagineers who are innovating in the world of beauty, science, technology, dermatology, and plastic surgery are all converging to create the longevity nation of healthy skin. In the future, more research, data, and the application of AI will lead to better treatments and products that will unveil themselves to the world. An important element of this will be ensuring widespread access to effective skincare. Democratizing the possibilities for every individual should be the goal, whether it is at a beauty counter, drugstore, doctor's office, or treatment center. Healthy skin, like a healthy body, should be for everyone.

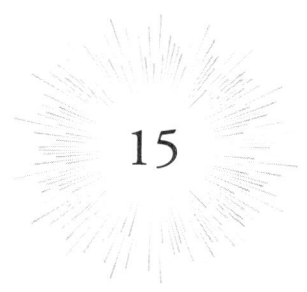

15

Relationships and Community Redefined for the Longevity Era

Loneliness. We all know it has become one of the chronic, debilitating issues of modern life. In a world of nearly 830 million people aged 65 or older, expecting to double to 1.7 billion by 2054, an aging population will be a growing societal issue for most developed nations.[1] In the US Surgeon General's 2023 advisory titled *Our Epidemic of Loneliness and Isolation*, it was reported that loneliness and social isolation are associated with a 26 percent and 29 percent increased risk of mortality, respectively.[2] A review published in *Nature Human Behaviour* found that social isolation was linked to a 32 percent higher risk of mortality.[3]

Loneliness can increase the risk of hypertension, heart disease, and stroke, as well as depression and anxiety.[4] While it can affect people of all ages, it is those over 65 who are the most vulnerable, as they step out of jobs and careers, lose spouses to divorce or death, and deal with families that have dispersed to other parts of the country or world.

In the era of longevity, how will people find ways to have social connections for longer, healthier lives?

Robert Waldinger, director of the Harvard Study of Adult Development, oversees the longest in-depth study of physical and mental well-being among adults. It has tracked hundreds of young adults from 1938 into their 80s.[5] Waldinger also cowrote the book *The Good Life: Lessons from the World's Longest Scientific Study of Happiness* with Marc Schulz. In an interview in the *Harvard Gazette*, Waldinger reported that satisfaction in relationships, particularly in marriages, was the best predictor of a happy and healthy life. He went on to say that the best data-backed hypothesis suggests that our relationships help us regulate stress. What he calls "social fitness" is as important as physical fitness and well-being when it comes to longevity.[6] He notes in the research that everybody needs at least one solid relationship. Who could you call in the middle of the night if you were sick or scared? Waldinger also points out that new relationships can start at any age, as our social life is a living system that relies on maintenance and ongoing cultivation. People at 70, 80, or older can make new friends of all ages. And in the future of the 100-year life, a new friendship at 70 could last thirty years!

In the 2020s, people have fewer institutional connections (like those formed through organized religion or affinity clubs) versus past generations. One benefit of those institutions was that they brought together people of all ages. Without them, people gravitate to others their own age who have had similar life experiences, which gives them a one-dimensional view of the world. In addition, large cohorts of older people either never married or are divorced or widowed. As of 2023, approximately 28 percent of Americans aged 50–64 and 36 percent of those aged 65 and older are single.[7] Among women aged 65 and older, 49 percent are single.

As we all live longer, the risk of loneliness and social isolation is poised to become an even bigger issue, especially for women. While there is increased awareness of the topic, who is focused on finding real-life solutions rather than just reporting on it? While it's important for researchers, doctors, sociologists, psychologists, the media, and others to highlight the concerns, where are the action plans to fix the problem?

Fortunately, there are initiatives around the world, fueled by organizations, nonprofits, local governments, and individuals, that are driving innovative approaches that will help those living longer lives. The efforts range from promoting multigenerational relationships to using new kinds of community groups, unique grassroots programs, and emerging technology to reduce loneliness. The people driving these ideas are the Re-Imagineers of community initiatives, and they are bringing people together in new ways.

Communities of All Kinds

In the city of Miami, Michael Roman is the community partnerships manager. He, along with others, led an initiative called EMPOWER60, which is designed to get people over 60 more involved in civic engagement.[8] When I asked Roman about the program in April 2025, he said, "We bring people together to teach them about their local government and then tap into them for what are they most passionate about, creating a civic engagement plan for them. For instance, if speeding on local streets is their issue, we might help them devise the approach to address it through a neighborhood resource officer or community meeting."[9]

Similar efforts have arisen around the country. For example, Seattle has created the Social Connectivity Learning Network for older adults to learn, share ideas, and collaborate for the betterment of their community, and Baltimore has created the Mayor's Office of Older Adults Affairs and Advocacy to include older adults to advise city leaders on how to make the community more age friendly. The Village to Village Network is a nonprofit that helps neighbors work together to allow aging at home, building community connections so people can lean on each other for friendship and support. The goal of Mirabella at Arizona State University is to foster intergenerational connections and community as part of everyday life.

Even if none of these specific groups are near you, a quick Google search is likely to turn up something similar centered around one of your interests. Finding groups of people who share your interests is one of the best proactive ways to build a community. I've done this myself. In this book, I previously wrote about my adventure travel group that has been in existence for more than twenty years. While we are all on a group chat to plot out our next adventure, we communicate with each other about life in general on an ongoing basis, acknowledging holidays and birthdays and planning other social get-togethers when we are not traveling. We've established a unique community around our shared passion for adventure travel, and

> **Finding groups of people who share your interests is one of the best proactive ways to build a community**

members of our group are always looking for new like-minded travelers who may be interested in what we do.

Just as it's beneficial to build social groups with people of mixed ages, it's also a good idea to include mixed genders. Many studies have found that women tend to be better at building and sustaining community than men. According to one of them, women share more openly with their friends and rely on friendships more often for social support, which has both physical and psychological benefits.[10] An article published by the Institute for Family Studies suggests that men have less experience communicating about their feelings, which hinders them from forming deep friendships.[11] Another study done by TheLi.st with the boutique ad agency Berlin Cameron and the research and strategy firm BSG revealed that 44 percent of men in corporate jobs say that being at work is the loneliest time of the day, and they are significantly less likely than women to turn to friends for support when they are facing challenges, particularly at work.[12]

Fortunately, new support groups are emerging to help men learn the kinds of skills they need to create communities and reduce loneliness, especially as they age. One such resource is MELD (Men's Emotional Leadership Development). Cofounder Owen Marcus says his approach, grounded in the latest scientific understanding of stress, trauma, and emotional physiology, offers a robust alternative to traditional models of men's emotional health. "One of the most groundbreaking aspects of our work is the emphasis on communal growth and connection. At the heart of our methodology is somatic mindfulness: the practice of using body awareness as a conduit for emotional awareness and expression," he explained in a 2024 article for ROAR forward.[13]

Sean Galla, who describes himself as founder and facilitator, has built a company called MensGroup, an online community for men that has dedicated support groups for divorce, infidelity, and more. "We've worked with thousands of guys and 92 percent of them have told us that they don't have any friends to talk to," he said.[14]

Groups such as Sacred Sons, ManKind Project, and EVRYMAN are other examples of ways for men to build community. The Midlife Male, founded by Re-Imagineer Greg Scheinman, includes content, community, and partnerships to help men at midlife come together to get insights, tips, and shared experiences from other men who are at the same stage of life, building lasting friendships and connections.

There are also approaches to building community that emphasize family and the value of pursuing multigenerational relationships. When my mother was in her mid-80s, she moved into an independent living complex near our family home. An active global traveler and someone who enjoyed being social with people of all ages, it took her only a few weeks to assess her new surroundings. "There are too many old people here who only talk about the past and complain about their aches and pains," she said to my brother Joe.[15]

While she had her children and grandchildren nearby, giving her exposure to multiple generations, many of her new neighbors weren't as fortunate. Many traditional independent living complexes, nursing homes, and age-restricted environments limit interactions to people who are the same age. This can exacerbate loneliness. How can we find new models and approaches to force change on the nursing home industry? Age segregation isn't healthy for anyone.

CoGenerate is an organization committed to bridging generational divides to cocreate the future. Marc Freedman and Eunice Lin Nichols are co-CEOs with a deep commitment to building cross-generational relationships. When I spoke with Freedman in March 2025, he explained why this was important: "The research shows that there is a complementarity of the assets of generations. I think this deep emotional longing to connect across generational lines to get a sense of the wholeness of life is very real."[16]

Age segregation isn't healthy for anyone

CoGenerate has given grants to multiple organizations that are working with people of all ages to find common ground and solutions. Freedman points out that there is also intergenerational richness in areas like music. Johnny Cash and Rick Rubin, Lady Gaga and Tony Bennett, Kris Kristofferson and Sinéad O'Connor, and Brandi Carlile and Elton John are just a few examples of pairings that have the potential to appeal to people of all generations, bringing them together in the shared experience of music. CoGenerate plans to launch

"Generations Got Talent" to promote the idea even further: "Imagine if we could create a crowdsourced cultural phenomenon that's built around the idea of what people across generations could do together in creating music."[17]

In a 2025 report entitled *Can Intergenerational Connection Heal Us?*, CoGenerate highlighted the critical role community organizations play in bringing generations together to reduce social isolation and loneliness. The report is a rich compendium on how small and hyper-local organizations are bringing older and younger people together for friendship, learning, collaboration, joy, and healing, listing more than 150 organizations committed to the idea. Examples include Mamaw Mentorship, a group in Central Appalachia created by Gwen Johnson to bring older women and girls in junior high school together to learn from each other. Hey Auntie! is a relationship-building service and community connecting Black women across all ages and life stages to build networks of friendships to help women thrive at home, at work, and in life. The Koreatown Storytelling Program in Los Angeles is designed to connect high school students and older people to tell their stories to each other and record them for their community.[18]

Dance may be another way to bring the generations together to form friendships and combat social isolation. Intergenerational Groove is organized by the NYC Department for the Aging, bringing people of all ages together to celebrate movement, music, and community.[19] More than a thousand participants join in every year for a day of social connection and well-being, creating new friendships as a byproduct of the festivities.

In my own family, we are intentional about making sure that all the generations come together on a regular basis to learn about our family history. Both of my paternal grandparents were Irish immigrants who came to America in the early twentieth century. One year, a multi-generational group of us went to County Monaghan to spend time with our large extended Irish family and to study the family tree, which was traceable back to 1791. Ranging in age from 3 to nearly 90, we shared stories, wisdom, and connections, all brought to life by our cousin Suzanne, the family historian, who had letters, photographs, and documents that chronicled our family's activities.

In 2024, when I visited Western Australia, I met Pat Torres, an elder in the Indigenous community near the city of Broome. At 70, she has committed herself to remembering and preserving the history and knowledge of the Djugun, Yawuru, and Karajarri groups she is descended from.[20] She studies the language and customs and has created the Jarndu Ngaank Tours not only to connect multiple generations from the Indigenous community, but to engage anyone who wants to learn more about Australia's early inhabitants. "My Djugun language community was based on the matrilineal knowledge systems of kinship, country, and a sense of belonging," she explained.[21]

Across the globe there are other inspiring grassroots initiatives finding new ways to address loneliness by bringing generations together.

Ole Kassow is a Danish social entrepreneur who founded the non-profit organization Cycling Without Age with a simple idea; younger and older people take a bicycle ride together, allowing them to create a sense of community as they share their stories. Created in Copenhagen in 2012, the program is now in forty-one countries.[22]

In Finland, homeshare programs match older homeowners with young people seeking affordable housing. A Home That Fits, launched in Helsinki, offers affordable studio apartments to young adults under twenty-five in older peoples' homes at reduced rates.[23] In exchange, the younger tenant agrees to spend three to five hours a week with the older neighbor, providing company and helping with everyday needs. A similar program called Nesterly has been launched in Boston. Humanitas in the city of Deventer in the Netherlands is another example.

The Dutch supermarket Jumbo introduced a "chat checkout" line to help fight loneliness among people in the communities they serve. This special, slower line allows people to take their time and have a conversation with one of the cashiers. It's augmented by an "All Together Coffee Corner" where people can sit and meet other locals and volunteers specifically for the purpose of social interaction.[24]

Sometimes the solutions are as simple as bringing people together in everyday interactions to stave off a sense of disconnection.

Sometimes the solutions are as simple as bringing people together in everyday interactions

Common themes in Asia include integrating care facilities and schools or daycare centers in the same building. Great examples include Shanghai's Sunshine Home, and St. Joseph's Home in Singapore. The natural connection among generations promotes relationships that combat social isolation and loneliness.

Building Connections Through Technology

While in-person connections are considered the best way to foster community, technology in all of its forms will become more and more relevant in the future. The solutions are already happening across the world in ways that will only accelerate, oftentimes driven by the wonders of AI. Examples include social connection platforms like Cyber-Seniors, which builds generational connections through technology training; Mon Ami, which connects seniors with college-age students; and Papa, which connects older adults with families who help with everyday tasks. Eldera connects younger people and older adults for shared experiences to create ongoing relationships, ensuring that conversations remain safe and supportive through the use of an AI chaperone. Virtual reality and digital experiences such as MyndVR, Rendever, and Wowzitude offer immersive experiences in travel and entertainment, a way for aging populations to combat loneliness, especially since many of the experiences are done in group settings.

With new technologies, caregivers may also be able to spend more quality time with those they care for. It is estimated that 41.8 million Americans are caring for individuals aged 50 and older.[25]

Weston Ballard is a new breed of longevity entrepreneur, using AI to support caregivers. After earning his MBA at the Stanford Graduate School of Business, Ballard launched Goldie in 2025 (see gotgoldie .com), a platform designed to empower modern emotional and social support facilitators, coaches, doulas, peer community leaders, and support group managers.[26] Goldie is an AI cofacilitator helping people run more impactful sessions while reducing their administrative burden. It helps plan sessions, match participants, lead empathetic voice AI check-ins, and more. Ultimately, it frees the facilitator to focus on connections instead of logistics: "With Goldie, we're elevating the human connection work that so much of our longevity depends on. Less burnout of facilitators means more support available to so many more people," Ballard said.[27]

Similar examples include Magnolia, an AI-first platform that integrates family caregivers in the United States into the healthcare system, and Wellthy, an employer-sponsored program that eases the burden on caregivers, allowing them to have more quality time with those they are caring for versus being mired in administrative tasks.

We're only at the beginning of how technology and AI will assist the community of caregivers. Robotics will be the next big frontier to create digital companions for all of us. While the idea seems daunting and provocative to some, there are AI-infused solutions that are already seeing positive results.

ElliQ is an AI Care Companion robot already in the marketplace as a tool to promote independence and healthy living.[28] Launched in the United States in 2022, it is primarily distributed to individuals by nonprofits, health plans, and governments at the state and county level to improve quality of

> **We're only at the beginning of how technology and AI will assist the community of caregivers**

life. An interactive desktop device that accumulates knowledge and behavior from interactions with a human, it is leading the way for the next generation of community: "While ElliQ is designed for people in their 60s or older, it's not about age, but rather about addressing loneliness. We have users from their 40s to our oldest user who is 103 years old," said Assaf Gad, vice president at the company.[29]

Gad reports that it's working well so far: "We call ElliQ a friendly robot, and 75 percent of our participants have told us that their social network has expanded due to its capabilities."[30]

A private company funded by a consortium of leading companies such as Toyota and Samsung, as well as venture capital groups, ElliQ is only available in the United States, but the company has global ambitions. According to Gad, they are also working on ways to connect it to a wearable device or smart TV in order to have broader accessibility, as well as integrating caregiving capabilities into the offering.

Other examples currently in the market include Pepper, a four-foot-tall humanoid robot created by SoftBank Robotics, and LOVOT, a home robot that creates emotional connections.

Ultimately, community through technology is going to take all kinds of forms. Who knows what will happen over the next years as digital and AI capabilities continue to evolve and new products are created. What we do know is that it will reimagine what community means.

The Longevity Nation Community

Although loneliness and isolation are major problems faced by many older adults, as we've discussed, there are solutions. Technology and AI will certainly help, but it will take more than that. In the longevity nation, the key is to find ways that work for everyone, regardless of who they are and where they live. As more and more people begin living to 100 or older, we'll need more support from governments, nonprofits, public-private partnerships, venture capital, and entrepreneurs to think about future solutions that will benefit everyone.

In the longevity nation, the key is to find ways that work for everyone, regardless of who they are and where they live

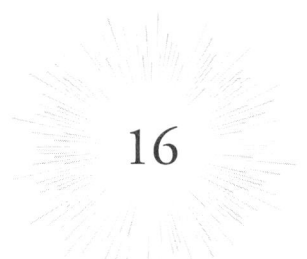

16

Here Comes the Longevity Neighborhood, Community, City, Country

One of the major trends to emerge in the longevity sphere is the desire to age in place. In response, governments, real estate developers, investors, technologists, and others are creating exciting new policies, models, and approaches that will provide housing options for people at all socioeconomics levels.

There has been an impressive amount of research, studies, and guidance from academic, nonprofit, and government organizations, providing the blueprints for getting the world "longevity ready." While many countries have already begun the process to adapt to this changing world, the United States, especially the federal government, continues to lag on awareness, policies in action, and funding versus what is happening in many parts of the world.

There is some progress being made, however. In 2017, the US Conference of Mayors established its Aging Task Force to address the reality that the number of older Americans will more than double over the next forty years, reaching 80 million in 2040.[1] In 2023, New York City introduced a resolution to promote age-inclusive cities, leading to the formation of a National Age-Inclusive Working Group comprising eighteen other US cities with older populations.

Despite this, there is still a lot of work to be done. Fortunately, there are a number of countries around the world whose example the United States can follow.

Singapore

When people ask me where they can find best practices for cities and communities that are driving a new longevity approach, my one-word answer is usually Singapore. As I've mentioned before, there is so much to learn from this tropical nation in Southeast Asia. Of its 3.64 million citizens, around 20 percent are 65 or older, and by 2030, that group is expected to grow to 24 percent.[2] Although even this projected percentage is lower than the percentage of the population that is 65 or older in Monaco (36 percent) and Japan (30 percent) today, Singapore has become a great role model on how to become a longevity nation.[3]

Let's start with the $3 billion (Singaporean dollars) Action Plan for Successful Ageing launched by the Ministerial Committee on Ageing in 2015. It's a national blueprint for everyone to age while maintaining active lives in an inclusive city for all.[4] Age Well SG was launched as a program to support living longer at home while ensuring social isolation is not a part of that experience.

I traveled to Singapore in 2024 to participate in the Milken Institute's Asia Summit, a phenomenal gathering of thought leaders from around the world who tackle some of the world's pressing issues. The Urban Redevelopment Authority is the national land use urban planning authority of Singapore, and one of their goals is to shape a happy, healthy city by working with partner government organizations to plan and design inclusive, connected, and accessible spaces that support active lifestyles and aging in place. The details are apparent as you walk around the city and see what has been done. Things like bold, colorful signage for directions, walkways and paths that incorporate physical and mental exercises, and therapeutic gardens that stimulate senses are just a few examples.

I learned at the conference that the national target is to have parks within a ten-minute walk of any apartment, use universal design elements in all public housing, and design new kinds of housing to accommodate the diverse preferences of an aging population, such as for multi-generational families called Three-Generation (3Gen) flats.

Redesigning public housing to be more age-inclusive will have a large impact in Singapore, since nearly 80 percent of residents live in these homes.[5]

But even better, Singapore is redesigning whole neighborhoods. "Self-contained towns" with coffee shops, restaurants, food stores, clinics, and other services within easy distance allows Singaporeans to age in place longer. Queenstown, the first satellite housing town in Singapore, is now being piloted as the city's first "Health District," creating age-friendly infrastructure and programs.[6] Other efforts include building a dementia-friendly neighborhood with six core principles that the Agency for Integrated Care developed to support the Ministry of Health's agenda on this front.

The Community for Successful Ageing (ComSA) is a program initiated by the Tsao Foundation in 2015, designed to help people age in place by integrating social services, healthcare, and well-being.[7] The foundation was established by Tsao Ng Yu Shun in 1993 as a nonprofit to enable older people to have a better quality of life. Today, the Foundation is overseen by her granddaughter, Dr. Mary Ann Tsao, and their programs have grown into sterling examples of longevity in action.

When I met Paul Ong, deputy CEO and chief strategy officer of the foundation, he explained that Singapore has reframed the issue from "aging" to "longevity," which underscores the more positive possibilities. "The goal of longevity here is that everything is predicated on a healthy life, which is physical, psychological, and environmental," he explained.[8]

In Singapore, it is a group effort to create one of the premier longevity cities in the world. The players include the government, public-private partnerships, nonprofits, academia, and more, all working in tandem for a common goal. For example MediSave, the national medical savings plan, has a Flexi-MediSave plan for Singaporeans over 60, who as of April 2025 can use up to S$300 of their accounts to cover outpatient expenses.[9] In 2023, Singapore launched a first-of-its-kind healthy longevity clinic in a public hospital, a collaboration between

> **it is a group effort to create one of the premier longevity cities in the world**

the National University Health System Centre for Healthy Longevity and Alexandra Hospital.

The list goes on and on with regard to the initiatives and innovations happening in Singapore in all sectors. My advice is that anyone who is interested in building the longevity city of the future should visit Singapore. Every elected official in the United States should go there for inspiration on what policies to enact on the local, state, and federal levels.

The United Arab Emirates

In 2024, development of the world's first city dedicated to longevity and wellness was announced: Longevi-City in Ras Al Khaimah, United Arab Emirates.[10] Dr. Raees Tonse, the driving force behind the project, said, "Longevi-City represents a movement towards a healthier future for all. By leveraging cutting-edge advances in healthcare, technology, and community development, it empowers individuals and communities to lead longer, healthier, and more fulfilling lives."[11]

One of the core efforts will be to give residents access to comprehensive healthcare services for optimized physical health, as well as mental and emotional well-being. Other elements include sustainable living and community engagement to foster healthy living practices. While there is no publicly announced completion date for Longevi-City, the world will be eagerly watching to learn and adapt best practices as they are created with this effort.

Japan

Japan has also developed new initiatives to adapt to its aging population—the highest proportion of older citizens in the world, according to the UN's report *World Population Ageing 2019*.[12] Cities like Fujisawa and Kashiwa-no-ha are being redesigned as age-friendly communities. Government programs such as Society 5.0 and the Smart Platinum Society don't just address the country's aging population needs but have a positive impact on all generations. Introduced by the Japanese government in 2016, Society 5.0 is the development of the "Super

Smart Society."[13] Identified as the fifth stage of societal evolution, the focus is on all things technology. According to the government report, the fusion of cyberspace and physical space and the values of a human-centered society will manifest this new environment. In the longevity space, it might include remote healthcare, care robots, monitoring systems, and data-driven wellness programs that are integrated into everyday life. One example is CareGo, which uses AI to detect changes in behaviors that might warrant health interventions. Key features include personalized care advisors, a resource hub, community support, human assistance, and technological tools to alleviate the challenges of caregiving.

In the city of Fujisawa, multiple initiatives include efforts to support aging in place with tech-enabled homes, eco-conscious living, and robotic assistance. The Shonan Robo Care Center is focused on how robotic devices can help to improve the mobility as their citizens live longer.[14]

Smart Platinum Society, created in 2015, was designed to encourage people to stay healthy and to continue to play active roles in both work and community during their robust 100-year life.[15] The government is implementing various measures to create what they call an "age-free" society in which people all of ages can thrive. With lower birthrates and fewer younger people, the country has focused on infrastructural issues like accessibility and walkability in reformatted urban planning initiatives. Sidewalks, universal design in public buildings, and transportation systems are just a few examples of creating a longevity nation. The Japanese government has also introduced universal access to home-based and institutional care for citizens 65 and older, allowing more people to stay in their homes and communities as they live longer.

Emi Kiyota is the founder of Ibasho, a nonprofit dedicated to cocreating socially integrated, sustainable communities that value their elders. The word *ibasho* means a place where one feels at home being oneself.[16] A Japanese national, Kiyota holds a PhD in architecture (environment and behavior) from the University of Wisconsin, as well as other degrees and fellowships. When I spoke with her in October 2024, she explained, "What I learned is that people who are over 65—

especially 65 to 70 years old—they are pretty healthy, they don't need care, and they want to do something to contribute back to the community. It was the big [lesson] as I set up the first program in Japan."[17]

> **they are pretty healthy, they don't need care, and they want to do something to contribute back to the community. It was the big [lesson] as I set up the first program in Japan**

An Ibasho community is economically, socially, and environmentally sustainable and is run by the community as a hub to make a difference. Kiyota has also established similar programs in Singapore, Nepal, and the Philippines. As a Re-Imagineer creating a new kind of model, she is helping us discover how we might live in different ways as we build a longevity nation.

Currently working as an associate professor at the National University of Singapore, Kiyota is also director of the Centre for Environment and Ageing Well, which explores new solutions for communities and cities, especially in Asia. "Many of the age-friendly city guidelines are created for Western [populations], but things are very different in the East. We are physically smaller; our lifestyles and family relations are different," she explained.[18] As a result, she is focusing on what aging in place can look like in the context of Asian communities, how people can adapt to change with different brain health issues, and how cities can build environments that address the issue of climate change, specifically with older citizens in mind.

The United Kingdom

Another major effort in how to build longevity cities is the UK National Innovation Centre for Ageing project. The city of Newcastle upon Tyne created the City of Longevity initiative and hosted the inaugural City of Longevity Global Conference in 2023, which brought together leaders from government, nonprofits, and multiple sectors of business.[19] One of the outcomes was the establishment of a comprehensive toolkit for local governments, planners, and policymakers to use in creating inclusive and accessible urban environments that support healthy aging. As part of the overall effort, Newcastle University is also developing the United Kingdom's first Health Innovation Neighbourhood on the former Newcastle General Hospital site. The effort aims to integrate housing, healthcare, and research facilities to create a model for holistic community well-being. It also plans to deliver high-value jobs and life-long learning opportunities within the complex.

Other Longevity Community Efforts

The initiatives in Singapore, the United Arab Emirates, Japan, and the United Kingdom are far from the only efforts to improve cities around the world in ways that promote and support longevity. Other examples include Barcelona's Superblocks program, which is working to reclaim public spaces for more walkable and greener urban areas; Geneva's Longevity Hub by Clinique La Prairie in Switzerland; and in South Korea, Seoul's 2020 Aging Society Master Plan, which is building a "healthy and lively city of citizens over age 100."[20]

Alana Officer is the unit head of Demographic Change and Healthy Ageing for the World Health Organization (WHO).[21] Based in Geneva, Switzerland, she and her colleagues coordinate the work for the UN Decade of Healthy Ageing, a ten-year initiative established by the United Nations (2021–2030). Aimed at improving the lives of the aging citizens of the 194 member countries and beyond, the focus is on age-friendly environments, combating ageism, and advocating for intergenerational connections. "The goal is to foster longer and healthier lives physically and mentally, allowing people to contribute, grow, and reinvent as they live longer lives," she said.[22]

Officer also oversees WHO's Global Network for Age-Friendly Cities and Communities (GNAFCC), which was founded in 2010 to help leaders find ways to adapt to their aging populations. "We currently have more than 1,600 cities and communities from fifty-two countries who are engaged on our age-friendly platform. It is a way to exchange information and experiences that support things like older people's inclusion and contributions to all areas of their lives," she said.[23]

Her predecessor, Dr. John Beard, currently the director of the International Longevity Center at Columbia University, played a key role in building out the network. "Today, more than three hundred million people are a part of the communities that are engaged in the work of the network. The diversity of needs are important. Older people are not a homogeneous group, they are incredibly diverse even within a given city. It's important to think about that with regard to their needs," he said."[24]

Beard believes that getting a city ready for older populations also has a benefit for younger populations, especially as they age—not to mention helping younger people with disabilities who might benefit from a more inclusive environment.

In the United States, the *Age-Inclusive American Cities Guidebook*, published in June 2024, identifies four action areas: deliberate communication, legislation, partnership, and design.[25] Some examples it explores include how cities and states can give incentives to businesses to partner on age-friendly initiatives, and how city planners, architects, zoning officials, and others can become part of an age-friendly task force.

Becoming a part of GNAFCC provides support and best practices to start the process whether you are an everyday citizen, city council member, or other elected official of any community, municipality, or neighborhood. Becoming an activist where you live will raise the awareness of the importance of moving this agenda forward.

In 2022, the World Bank Group published *Silver Hues: Building Age-Ready Cities*, which suggested that we should make our cities future-ready by proactively thinking about and investing intentionally in planning and designing for the longevity of people.[26] The six key principles in the report are universal design, age-ready housing solutions, access to multigenerational spaces and activities, easy transportation capabilities, technology enablers, and efficient spatial forms (the idea of the fifteen-minute city with everything that is needed within that walkable radius).

Re-Imagineers have created an amazing number of reports, analyses, and pathways for countries to begin the process of becoming longevity friendly. If you are interested in identifying which countries have been the best at it, you may want to learn about the John A. Harford Foundation Aging Society Index, produced by the Research Network on an Aging Society. Made up of a fourteen-member disciplinary group of demographers, sociologists, psychologists, policy experts, and more, the network formulated an evidence-based model of a success-ful aging society that leads to better longevity. The study assessed the status of older populations across five specific domains: productivity and engagement, well-being, equity, economic and physical security, and intergenerational cohesion. Using data from the Organisation for Economic Co-operation and Development (OECD), WHO, and other sources, each domain had a weighting from 17 to 25 percent (well-being being the highest with healthy life expectancy and life satisfaction for those 50 and older).[27] While Japan ranked the highest in well-being due to healthy life expectancies there, the United States ranked number one in productivity due to high effective retirement age and high rates of volunteerism. Overall, the number one ranked country was Norway, followed by Sweden and then the United States, the Netherlands, and Japan, with all of them still having room for improvement. While this is only one study, it is a great barometer of the kinds of measures that governments and policymakers need to pay attention to for future success.

The Situation in the United States

As previously mentioned, the United States has a lot of catching up to do with regard to its own aging population. Topics such as infrastructure, design, legislation, and partnerships are all relevant to getting the country longevity ready. It can happen at the federal, state, or local levels and should include players from all sectors in the commercial world. Real estate developers, technologists, and private equity can all have a part in creating a new future in how we will live. Investing in this (literal) space will provide great returns and profits.

the United States has a lot of catching up to do

Major cities with more than 20 percent of their populations age 60 and older include Miami (26.1 percent), Albuquerque (22.6 percent), San Francisco (22.5 percent), and New York (21 percent).[28] Smaller cities like Scottsdale (24.6 percent) and Honolulu (20.5 percent) are also part of the growing ranks of Americans who are living longer.[29]

However, although the United States lags behind many developed nations in its efforts to accommodate a longevity lifestyle, some key people are working to close that gap. One of these is Ryan Frederick, who is what I call a Re-Imagineer leader, with an intent to create real-life solutions for the next generation of housing to let people thrive in the second half of their lives, regardless of what city they live in. A speaker and strategy consultant in the real estate and healthcare sectors, he is also the author of *Right Place, Right Time: The Ultimate Guide to Choosing a Home for the Second Half of Life*. After the book was published, he started the company Here, the home of Place Planning. "There is a gap in the market between when one wants to transition from single family housing and the leap into what has been a restricted age, senior living, or retirement community," he said.[30]

Frederick believes that while those might be options for some, many healthy, vibrant people over 50 don't want that kind of living experience. He sees a major trend in people choosing to buy or rent in places that fit this new period in their lives with a different set of criteria that might include interactions with people of all ages, different kinds of social programming, and access to more amenities. His philosophy is that an individual or couple should be "place planning" the same way that they focus on financial or health planning, because "a misalignment on what your needs are now and where you live can impact you in a negative way."[31]

His online assessment tool at www.here.life allows people to assess four dimensions (environment, health, community, and finances) to explore what might be right for them. Ultimately, someone may determine that staying in a house in the suburbs where they raised their kids is no longer relevant to them. Frederick is changing the conversation by guiding users through a deep process of understanding what is important to them now. He has also identified some examples of new models that are emerging to capitalize on different kinds of living choices for those in the second half of life. For example, the Stories at Congressional Plaza in Rockville, Maryland, has built units with longevity in mind: "It is not overly obvious, but there are slip-resistant tiles on the floor, easy-to-use levers, showers not bathtubs, and more.

People can live there longer, as what they need as they age is already in the design," he explained.[32]

Other examples include the build-for-rent (BFR) model for those who don't want to commit to buying another home, accessible dwelling units (ADUs) for those who have mobility or sensory limitations, and apartment buildings that are intentionally created as NORCs (naturally occurring retirement communities). There is also a new movement for more multi-generational housing, an effort that Lennar Builders is leading, according to Frederick. To raise awareness of the importance of this new segment and their desire to not necessarily move into an age-restricted building or over-55 community, Frederick has created Certified Place Planners to help real estate agents and wealth advisors guide their clients into many of these new options.

Throughout the country, there are new models emerging to satisfy what is going to be a very diversified population of older people with different ideas about how they want to live as they live longer. Long gone are the days when the only option is to move into an adult community, the Villages in Florida, or a traditional retirement development. People thriving in the second half of life are creating all kinds of new living experiences.

They include Urbaneer, founded by Bruce Thompson with a goal to develop an ageless design approach that combines smart home and wellness technologies, and the Green House Project, an alternative to the traditional nursing home model that creates small, intentional communities of ten to twelve older individuals who support each other. With longer, healthier lives, we are watching people completely rethink how they will live.

Other options may be found internationally. For example, my friend Peri and her husband, Charlie, both in their 80s, are building a new home in Mexico. My friends Lori and Jerry, both in their 60s, have chosen to become expats in Portugal.

Some residences are super-high-end urban luxury apartment buildings with built-in medical services, gourmet dining, and world class speakers and activities, like Coterie Hudson Yards and Inspīr Carnegie Hill in New York City. When I visited both, it was clear that this was not your typical "senior housing" but rather beautifully designed buildings and units that are hi-tech enabled and filled with vibrant occupants. Other high-end places include Vi at Palo Alto and the Variel in Woodland Hills, California.

New options will also include cohousing, where family and friends get together to share a compound or become roommates who support each other over their longer lives. My friends Emily and Bill, who live in New Mexico, have the idea to build a main compound surrounded by smaller units that belongs to friends, creating the twenty-first century version of a commune.

All of these options are designed to allow people to live longer in a new place of their choice. It's a new form of housing activism.

One of my favorite new longevity housing models is Mirabella at Arizona State University, which just might be the template for an entirely new type of living for people over 50. Situated on campus, Mirabella residents receive a university ID and have complete access to all facilities, as well as the ability to audit classes. Unlike other university-affiliated residential communities (which can be found on UniversityRetirementCommunities.com), Mirabella is uniquely embedded into everyday life on the campus, resulting in organic intergenerational engagement.

According to Lindsey Beagley, the senior director of Lifelong University Engagement for Mirabella, residents find themselves creating relationships with faculty, university employees, and students of all ages. "The majority of our residents are in their 70s and are well-educated. Eighty percent have master's degrees and are very engaged. I'd call them a campus adventurer," she explained, adding that "the University's commitment to the project also brings insights into how older adults want to learn."[33]

Mirabella has more than three hundred residents, but only 17 percent are alumni. The majority were attracted to both the model and the Arizona climate, according to Beagley.

She also points to South Korea as a country that is focused on a similar approach. "We've had seven or eight Korean universities come to visit us. They've also created an inter-university coalition called UBRC Korea to learn from each other," she explained.[34] In order to elevate and expand the model in the United States, Beagley and others are working on the first longevity innovation and higher education summit, under the auspices of the Age-Friendly University Global Network.

Regardless of which additional models emerge, all of them will be enabled by new technologies that are already in existence or being created. Whether it is tele-medicine, sensor systems, robotics, or yet-to-be-introduced AI products for a smarter home, they are all designed to help people live a healthier life in the place that is best for them.

In a 2025 *New York Times* article entitled "Invasion of the Home Humanoid Robots," the writer Cade Metz reports that dozens of companies are building robots to move into our homes to help with daily chores. According to Metz, investments in the category hit $1.6 billion in 2024.[35] While it may be reminiscent of Rosie the Robot in the 1960s television series *The Jetson*s, it's not such a far-off idea to imagine how this might become a real product in the years to come.

New York state has one of the most ambitious initiatives, with more than twenty public-private partnerships with leading agetech innovators that support living in place.[36] Some of the digital or virtual tools include Team Vivo, an evidence-based strength training and exercise program; Emerest Connect, which provides 24/7 on-call nursing assistance; and GetSetUp, a discovery platform with more than five thousand courses in forty categories, including cybersecurity, technology, and more.

As the commissioner of the New York City Department for the Aging, Lorraine Cortés-Vázquez is leading the quest to make New York the most age-friendly city in America. "By 2030, all New York City neighborhoods will be naturally occurring retirement communities. They're all going to have more than 20 percent of their populations be of retirement age," she declared.[37]

Today, New York's 55-and-older residents make up 27 percent of the population (more than 2.3 million people), and Cortés-Vázquez is constantly thinking about ways to make the city better equipped.[38] While there are infrastructure issues like a lack of walkways and ramps, there is also the cost of housing, accessibility to transportation, the need for caregivers, and more. As a leading Re-Imagineer in government, in 2022, she convened twenty-four separate city agencies called the Cabinet for Older New Yorkers to see how they might work together to create solutions. One example has been the implementation of street audits, where a team from the Department of Transportation tours a neighborhood with a group of older adults. "They serve almost as the consultants to the engineers and then that gets incorporated into the early designs. They walk around and they experience the crosswalks and the lights and things with them," she explained.[39]

In 2024, she and First Deputy Commissioner/Chief Operating Officer Michael Ognibene hosted a first-of-its-kind conference called Boom! A Silver Dawning in American Cities. They invited representatives from eighteen other American cities, as well as other longevity-focused professionals, to share best practices and learn from one another on how best to address longer-living populations. As a participant in the conference, I was inspired to learn, for example, how Oklahoma City instituted a 1 percent tax dedicated to benefiting older adults there. Cortés-Vázquez's department has a wide variety of activities throughout the city, from hosting seventeen citywide town halls for older adults to launching a Service Needs Assessment Survey to gather input for policies and programs that will be relevant to a population that is living longer. They also fund programs to reduce costs on essentials such as food, health, transportation, and housing.

The new City of Yes program, passed by the City Council of New York, is an ambitious rezoning program that aims to expand housing opportunities throughout the city. As the plan states, the goal is to enable the creation of eighty-two thousand homes over the next fifteen years.[40] Cortés-Vázquez is in the middle of discussions on how this can bring more affordable housing to both older adults and caregivers across the city's five boroughs.

Longevity-Friendly Environments Are the Future

We are in an incredible moment of reinvention, as the more progressive and innovative countries, states, and municipalities build, reformat, and pay attention to the importance of longevity-friendly environments. For those who have an action plan, it will lead to better communities of happier and healthier people, attract economic investments for growth, and more.

Becoming known as a longevity city is the future currency for being known as a place where people of all ages want to live. It will benefit people of all ages, especially as the next generations move into this phase of their lives and drive economic growth for the towns and cities that focus on these efforts.

it will lead to better communities of happier and healthier people, attract economic investments for growth, and more

Conclusion

As we create the longevity nation of the future, the priority has to be ensuring that all the astounding developments in medicine, technology, and more are democratized and become available to everyone. It should be the global agenda for all of us as we prepare our children for a different kind of second half of life, filled with many new possibilities. It means governments will have to fund new initiatives, new public-private partnerships will need to be developed, and corporations and nonprofits will be obligated to step up to help in bigger ways.

Throughout this book, I've introduced you to many individuals who are reimagining a different future in medicine, technology, higher education, and more. They are joined by activists like Ashton Applewhite, the author of *This Chair Rocks: A Manifesto Against Ageism* and a cofounder of the Old School Hub, a grassroots organization for age equity and ageism awareness.[1] Louise Aronson, an American geriatrician and professor of medicine at the University of San Francisco, is the author of *Elderhood: Redefining Aging, Transforming Medicine, Reimagining Life*. Her central thesis is that society and the medical system need a paradigm shift for older adults.[2] Journalist Richard Eisenberg specializes in new ways to look at aging and living longer, helping change the narrative for what will be the remarkable realization of the 100-year life.

Peter Kaldes is a longtime nonprofit leader and currently the president and CEO of Next50, a Colorado-based private, national foundation with a mission to promote independence and dignity for the aging population. Their key initiatives include ending ageism, advancing digital equity, and supporting aging in place for everyone. "We are one of a handful of national foundations with a commitment to this sector. Only 1 to 2 percent of all philanthropic dollars are committed to aging," he explained.[3] Next50, the John A. Hartford Foundation, the RRF Foundation for Aging, the SCAN Foundation, and the AARP Foundation are examples of organizations that commit grants to the aging sector, but there needs to be more. With the billions being committed to drugs for longevity, where is the funding for other aspects of living better and longer lives?

According to Kaldes, there are corporations that do one-off sponsorships for conferences or fund a research project, but there is no ongoing commitment from the business community.[4] It's a big opportunity for corporate leaders to become a part of the longevity agenda.

With the billions being committed to drugs for longevity, where is the funding for other aspects of living better and longer lives

On the state and local levels, there are community-based efforts, along with private donors in towns and cities, but the need is for big dollars moving into the space to support housing, healthcare, and wellness, and caregiving for what will be eighty million people over 65 by the year 2040.[5]

Nationally, there are organizations such as the National Council on Aging, the Leadership Council of Aging Organizations, the American Society on Aging, and the National Institute on Aging, but they all rely on funding to support advocacy efforts and deliver on their missions to build a stronger future for older citizens in the United States. On the federal level, the National Institute on Aging has been a grantor for aging research and initiatives, but many of the programs have been shut down due to budget cuts. There's no real national political agenda to address the issues of an aging America, according to Kaldes.[6]

To address this deficit, Next50 recently announced that it will align its entire $270 million endowment with its mission by investing in various thematic portfolios supporting aging. "Our new portfolio will invest in creating economic opportunity, supporting the built environment, ensuring health, and expanding social inclusion," said Kaldes. "We have partnered with JPMorgan Chase to work with us on finding the right investments. A commitment from one of the leading banks in this space is a big step forward."[7]

But the agenda to build a longevity nation will also require the collective efforts of individuals from all over the world, and not just those we've discussed in this book. Those of us over 50 can harness our experience, knowledge, resources, and contacts to be the ones who may realize the 100-year life, but we should have a bigger legacy in mind. How do we get our children and their children ready for a radically different world where longevity may extend beyond a 100-year life? This may be the most important thing we do, not just for ourselves and our families but for the future of the world's population.

we should have a bigger legacy in mind

We can all play our part, at work, at home, and with our families and communities to create the longevity nation of today and the future.

Acknowledgments

The idea of *Longevity Nation* came together as I met incredible individuals who were all working on a common goal: to find solutions for all people to live longer, healthier lives for as long as possible. Many of them believe that the 100-year life is already here and will become more normalized in years to come.

There are so many people to thank who enabled me to tell the stories about the people, ideas, and trends that will change the second half of our lives. A special thanks to Michele and Richard Cohn, Linda Konner, Lindsay Easterbrooks-Brown, Sarah Heilman, Ashley Van Winkle, Karen Chernyaev, Brennah Hermo, Emmalisa Sparrow Wood, and the teams at Beyond Words, Atria, and Simon & Schuster.

A special thanks to Fran Crane, my colleague of forty years who keeps me on track in so many ways.

To Ken Bronfin at Hearst Ventures who has believed in the mission of ROAR forward since the beginning. I'm grateful for his support and guidance.

Also, a special thank you to Laura Carstensen PhD, founding director of the Stanford Center on Longevity who has been my friend and mentor throughout this project and more.

For those who shared their knowledge, experience, and wisdom, thanks to:

Celine
  Abecassis-Moedas
Ashton Applewhite
Amy Baer
Weston Ballard
Cyrus Bamji
Lindsay Beagley
John Beard
Luciano Bernardini
Melissa Biggs Bradley
Justin Boxford
Mark Buchanan
Dan Buettner
John-Morgan Bush
Laura Carstensen
Simon Chan
Anne Chang
Wendy Chapman
Barbara Chuback
Susan Lee Colby
Chip Conley
Tara Connaughton
Pamela Corante
Lynne Corner
Lorraine
  Cortés-Vásquez
Sara Czaja
Steve Dayan
Kevin Delaney
Manjit Devgun
John Dick
Annette Dunleavy
Richard Eisenberg
Diane Epstein
Michele Evans
Tamsen Fadal

Jason Fichtner
Jonathan Fisher
Ryan Frederick
Michael Fredericson
Marc Freedman
Linda Fried
Assaf Gad
Jonathan Gal
Jennifer Garrison
Laurie Gerber
Jenna Glover
Klara Glowczewski
Seth Green
David Greenberg
Tom Hale
Ei Phyo Han
Kerry Hannon
David Harris
Russ Hill
Dana Hilmer
Haideh Hirmand
Mafalda Honorio
Paul Irving
Louis Island
Mark T. Johnsen
Peter Kaldes
Stephanie Katz
Emi Kiyota
John Kneapler
Katy Knox
Barbara Kotlikoff
Stephanie Kramer
Erica Kwok
Vania Lacascade
Mark Lachs
Ruth La Ferla

Christopher Leech
Ben Legg
Abby Levy
Jane Lodato
Don Loftus
Valter Longo
David Luu
Craig Lyman
Gabrielle Lyon
Joan MacDonald
Andrea Maier
Mike Mansfield
Owen Marcus
Jeanne Marin
Debbie Marshall
Alison Matz
Patrick McCleary
Martha McCully
Norman Miller
Tim Minnick
Ron Minutella
Valerie Monroe
James Moses
Ronjon Nag
Sara Nasserzadeh
Haleh Nazeri
Phil Newman
Jeanne Noonan
Alana Officer
Michael Ognibene
Paul Ong
David Pagano
Jennifer Palmer
Peg Pardini
Sharon Parish
Alan Patricof

Alister Punton
René Quashie
Zakia Rahman
Alissa Randall
Tom Rando
Renee Rogers
Michael Roman
Alex Rotas
Jack Rowe
David Sable
Ebenezer Samuel
Steve Samuels
Katherine H.
   Saunders
Kate Schaefers

Jennifer Schrack
Bradley Schurman
Andrew Scott
Kerry Sette
Gopi Shah Goda
Yochai Z. Shavit
Steve Sharp
Lyndsey Simpson
Meeta Singh
Yvonne Sonsino
Don Spradlin
Emerson Sprick
Leslie Stevens
Mitchell Stevens
Yolanda Taylor

Paul Theroux
Diane Ty
Eric Verdin
Anh Vu Sawyer
Anthony Wagner
Barbara Waxman
Adam Weiss
Eric Williamson
Avivah
   Wittenberg-Cox
Tina Woods
Paul Woolmington
Wendy Wright

To the ROAR forward team, thanks for your enthusiasm and contributions to all things longevity.

Giulio Capua
Kathy DiBenedetto
Bill Gibbons
Beth Jacobson
Hillary Koota

Jennifer Lanzarone
Linda Mason
Ellen Oppenheim
Cara Deoul Perl
Kelly Peterson

Elisa Shevitz
Chris Tosti
Sean Walsh

Many in my professional Hearst family have supported my efforts from the beginning and continue to be interested in the work of ROAR forward. Thanks to Will Hearst III, Frank Bennack, Mary Lake Polan, Steve Swartz, Jordan Wertlieb, Mitch Scherzer, David Carey, Rachel Kay, Debi Chirichella, Maria Walsh, Victoria Pavlov, Alex Carlin, Gayle King, Hillary Koota, Lucy Kaylin, Richard Dorment, Abby Cuffey, Ben Court, Michael Sebastian, Stellene Volandes, Stephanie Dolgoff, Brian O'Keefe, Maureen Sheehan, Barb Maushard, Frank Biancuzzo, Lori Waldon, and many more.

To my family and friends, I'm forever grateful for their ongoing support. Their encouragement and curiosity have been the energy source that kept me going. A special thank you to Dr. Tom DeVincentis, who has been there every step of the way and knows a bit about longevity. To Chris Shirley, Dr. Keith LaScalea, and my sister Chris Evans who checked in regularly on the book's progress. Finally, to my dad Joseph, who passed away at 92 during the writing of this book. He and my late mom, Nancy, were always my biggest supporters. Their love taught me that all things are possible.

Recommended Books

Throughout this book, I share some of my favorite authors and books that have inspired me and given me insight into living a life that ROARs. Here is a list of all those titles. Happy reading!

Ageless: The New Science of Getting Older Without Getting Old by Andrew Steele (Doubleday, 2021)

Age Later: Health Span, Life Span, and the New Science of Longevity by Nir Barzilai (St. Martin's Press, 2020)

Aging While Black, A Radical Reimagining of Aging and Race in America by Raymond A. Jetson (Manuscripts Press, 2025)

Becoming Ageless: The Four Secrets to Looking and Feeling Younger Than Ever by Strauss Zelnick and Zack Zeigler (Galvanized Media, 2018)

Breaking the Age Code: How Your Beliefs About Aging Determine How Long and Well You Live by Becca Levy (William Morrow, 2022)

Elderhood: Redefining Aging, Transforming Medicine, Reimagining Life by Louise Aronson (Bloomsbury Adult, 2021)

How to Live Forever: The Enduring Power of Connecting the Generations by Marc Freedman (PublicAffairs, 2018)

How To Menopause: Take Charge of Your Health, Reclaim Your Life, and Feel Even Better than Before by Tamsen Fadal (Balance, 2025)

Ikigai: The Japanese Secret to a Long and Happy Life by Héctor Garcia and Francesc Miralles (Penguin Life, 2017)

In Control at 50+: How to Succeed in the New World of Work by Kerry Hannon (McGraw Hill, 2022)

Learning to Love Midlife: 12 Reasons Why Life Gets Better with Age by Chip Conley (Little, Brown Spark, 2024)

Longevity Guidebook: How to Slow, Stop, and Reverse Aging—and NOT Die from Something Stupid by Peter H. Diamandis (Ethos Collective, 2025)

Mindfulness for Beginners: Reclaiming the Present Moment—and Your Life by Jon Kabat-Zinn (Sounds True, 2016)

Much More to Come: Lessons on the Mayhem and Magnificence of Midlife by Eleanor Mills (HQ, 2025)

Optimizing Longevity: A Road Atlas for a Happier, Less Predictable Life by Russell T. Hill (Longevity Action Publishing, 2024)

Outlive: The Science and Art of Longevity by Peter Attia and Bill Gifford (Harmony, 2023)

Portfolio Life: The New Path to Work, Purpose, and Passion After 50 by David Corbett and Richard Higgins (John Wiley & Sons, Inc., 2007)

Sleep Clocks in Aging and Longevity edited by Anita Jagota (Springer, 2023)

The Sleep Revolution: Transforming Your Life, One Night at a Time by Arianna Huffington (Harmony Books, 2017)

Sleep Smarter: 21 Essential Strategies to Sleep Your Way to a Better Body, Better Health, and Bigger Success by Shawn Stevenson (Rodale, 2016)

The Great Money Reset: Change Your Work, Change Your Wealth, Change Your Life by Jill Schlesinger (St. Martin's Press, 2023)

The 100-Year Life: Living and Working in an Age of Longevity by Lynda Gratton and Andrew J. Scott (Bloomsbury Publishing, 2017)

The Longevity Diet: Slow Aging, Fight Disease, Optimize Weight by Valter Longo (Avery, 2019)

The Longevity Economy: Unlocking the World's Fastest-Growing, Most Misunderstood Market by Joseph F. Coughlin (PublicAffairs, 2017)

The Longevity Paradox: How to Die Young at a Ripe Old Age by Steven Gundry (Harper Wave, 2019)

The New Aging: Politics and Change in America by Fernando M. Torres-Gil (Auburn House, 1992)

The Singularity Is Nearer: When We Merge with AI by Ray Kurzweil (Viking, 2024)

The Super Age: Decoding Our Demographic Destiny by Bradley Schurman (Harper Business, 2022)

This Chair Rocks: A Manifesto Against Ageism by Ashton Applewhite (Networked Books, 2016)

What Your Doctor Won't Tell You About Getting Older: An Insider's Survival Manual for Outsmarting the Health-Care System by Mark Lachs (Penguin, 2011)

Why We Can't Sleep: Women's New Midlife Crisis by Ada Calhoun (Grove Press, 2020)

Why We Sleep: Unlocking the Power of Sleep and Dreams by Matthew Walker (Scribner, 2017)

Younger Next Year: Live Strong, Fit, Sexy, and Smart—Until You're 80 and Beyond by Chris Crowley and Henry S. Lodge (Workman Publishing, 2019)

Notes

Foreword

1. Thomas Hobbes, *Leviathan or the Matter, Forme, and Power of a Common-Wealth Ecclesiastical and Civil* (London, 1651), chap. 13, https://www.plato-philosophy.org/wp-content/uploads/Thomas-Hobbes-Leviathan-Chapter-13.pdf.

Preface

1. Tristan McConnell, "Today's 5-Year-Olds Will Likely Live to 100. What Will Their Lives Be Like?" *National Geographic*, February 24, 2023, https://www.nationalgeographic.com/magazine/article/half-of-todays-5-year-olds-will-live-to-be-100.
2. Department of Economic and Social Affairs Population Division, *World Population Prospects* 2024 (United Nations, 2024), https://population.un.org/wpp/.
3. Elizabeth Arias and Jiaquan Xu, "United States Life Tables, 2018," *National Vital Statistics Reports* 69, no. 12 (2020): table 13, https://stacks.cdc.gov/view/cdc/97643.
4. "Population Statistics," AARP, accessed September 26, 2025, https://datastories.aarp.org/the-lived-experience-of-adults-50-plus/population-statistics/index.html.
5. Ray Kurzweil, *The Singularity Is Nearer: When We Merge with AI* (Viking, 2024).

Introduction

1. ROAR forward and National Research Group, "Meet the Re-Imagineers," paper presented to ROAR clients, Fall 2023.
2. Employee Benefit Research Institute & Greenwald Research, "2024 RCS Fact Sheet #2: Expectations About Retirement," 2024, https://www.ebri.org/docs/default-source/rcs/2024-rcs/rcs_24-fs-2.pdf.
3. ROAR forward and National Research Group, "Meet the Re-Imagineers."
4. *The Graduate*, directed by Mike Nichols (1967, Lawrence Turman Productions), DVD, 43:33.

Chapter 1: The OG Re-Imagineers of Longevity

1. Laura Carstensen (professor, Stanford), in discussion with author, March 20, 2025.
2. Carstensen, discussion.
3. Carstensen, discussion.
4. "The OCS Study," Okinawa Research Center for Longevity Science, accessed September 28, 2025, https://www.orcls.org/ocs/.
5. Jack Rowe (professor, Columbia University), in discussion with author, April 11, 2025.
6. Rowe, discussion.
7. Rowe, discussion.
8. Linda Fried (dean, Columbia University), in discussion with author, January 28, 2025.
9. Fried, discussion.
10. Fried, discussion.
11. Fried, discussion.
12. Katherine Schaeffer, *U.S. Centenarian Population Is Projected to Quadruple over the Next 30 Years* (Pew Research Center, 2024), https://www.pewresearch.org/short-reads/2024/01/09/us-centenarian-population-is-projected-to-quadruple-over-the-next-30-years/.
13. "Lynne Corner," National Innovation Centre Ageing, accessed September 24, 2025, https://uknica.co.uk/blog/people/lynne-corner/.
14. Lynne Corner (COO, UK National Innovation Centre for Ageing), in discussion with author, October 22, 2024.
15. Corner, discussion.

16. Dan Buettner, "The Secrets of Long Life," *National Geographic*, November 2005, https://www.bluezones.com/wp-content/uploads/2015/01/Nat_Geo _LongevityF.pdf.

17. Dan Buettner (*Blue Zones* author), in discussion with author, April 4, 2025.

18. Buettner, discussion.

19. Buettner, discussion.

20. Buettner, discussion.

21. Paul Irving (senior advisor, Center for the Future of Aging), in discussion with author, February 20, 2025.

22. Irving, discussion.

23. Irving, discussion.

24. Diane Ty (managing director, Center for the Future of Aging), in discussion with author, March 3, 2025.

25. Andrew Scott, *The Longevity Imperative: How to Build a Healthier and More Productive Society to Support Our Longer Lives* (Basic Books, 2024).

26. Andrew Scott (professor, London Business School), in discussion with author, April 2, 2025.

27. Scott, discussion.

Chapter 2: New Personas for a Longevity Nation

1. Susan L. Brown and I-Fen Lin, "The Graying of Divorce: A Half Century of Change," *The Journals of Gerontology: Series B*, vol. 77, no. 9 (2022): 1710–20, https://academic.oup.com/psychsocgerontology/article/77/9/1710/6564346.

2. Elliott Jaques, "Death and the Mid-life Crisis," *International Journal of Psycho-Analysis* 46, no. 4 (1965): 502–514, https://pubmed.ncbi.nlm.nih.gov /5866085/.

3. Michael Clinton, *ROAR: into the second half of your life (before it's too late)*, Atria Books/Beyond Words, 2021.

4. Modern Elder Academy, "Your Best Years Are Ahead of You," accessed March 7, 2025, https://www.meawisdom.com/.

5. Patrick McCleary, in discussion with author, February 7, 2025.

6. McCleary, discussion.

7. McCleary, discussion.

8. Don Spradlin, in discussion with author, February 10, 2025.

9. Spradlin, discussion.

10. Spradlin, discussion.

11. Barbara Waxman (founder, Odyssey Group), in discussion with author, February 5, 2025.

12. Waxman, discussion.

13. Waxman, discussion.

14. Chip Conley, "The Gift of Cancer (Part 1)," *Wisdom Well* (blog), Modern Elder Academy, November 18, 2024, https://www.meawisdom.com/the-gift-of-cancer-part-1/.

15. Michele Evans (founder, NxtWaves), in discussion with author, August 30, 2024.

16. Mark Buchanan, in discussion with author, February 7, 2025.

17. Buchanan, discussion.

18. Buchanan, discussion.

19. Aaron Hicklin, "David Bowie: An Obituary," *Out Magazine*, January 11, 2016, https://www.out.com/music/2016/1/11/david-bowie-obituary.

20. Dana Hilmer (cofounder, Camp Reinvention), in discussion with author, December 24, 2024.

21. Hilmer, discussion.

22. Pamela Corante, in discussion with author, February 10, 2025.

23. Corante, discussion.

24. Corante, discussion.

25. Corante, discussion.

26. Corante, discussion.

27. Hilmer, discussion.

Chapter 3: Lifelong Learning: Should You Go Back to School to Relaunch Your Life?

1. Saleen Martin, "90-Year-Old Who Got Degree After 'Many' All-Nighters Has 'a Lot of Good Living Left to Do,'" *USA Today*, December 21, 2023, https://www.usatoday.com/story/life/humankind/2023/12/21/minnie-payne-90-north-texas/71982583007/.

2. "Oldest Graduate," Guinness World Records, accessed February 7, 2025, https://www.guinnessworldrecords.com/world-records/oldest-graduate.

3. Avivah Wittenberg-Cox, "Aging Relevantly: Getting Good at Midlife Transitions," *Forbes*, July 25, 2021, https://www.forbes.com/sites/avivahwittenbergcox/2021/07/25/aging-relevantly-getting-good-at-midlife-transitions/.

4. U.S. Fish and Wildlife Service, "Theodore Roosevelt (1858–1919) the Conservation President," accessed February 7, 2025, https://www.fws.gov/staff-profile/theodore-roosevelt-1858-1919-conservation-president.

5. Theodore Roosevelt, "The Strenuous Life," speech delivered at the Hamilton Club, Chicago, April 10, 1899, transcript, Theodore Roosevelt Association, https://www.theodoreroosevelt.org/content.aspx?page_id=22&club_id=991271&module_id=339361.

6. Michael Clinton, "A Social Entrepreneur Is Born at Age 67," *Oprah Daily*, November 3, 2023, https://www.oprahdaily.com/life/work-money/a45726344/anh-vu-sawyer-social-entrepreneur/.

7. Clinton, "Social Entrepreneur."

8. Clinton, "Social Entrepreneur."

9. David Harrison, in discussion with author, September 8, 2024.

10. Rebecca Mathews, Bijan Warner, and Peter Stokes, "Managing the Demand Cliff," *Inside Higher Ed*, October 16, 2023, https://www.insidehighered.com/opinion/views/2023/10/16/managing-other-enrollment-cliff-opinion.

11. Louis Island (physiotherapist), in discussion with the author, September 24, 2024.

12. Jeanne Marin (dermatologist and surgeon), in discussion with the author, February 10, 2025.

13. Marin, discussion.

14. Kate Schaefers (director, Osher Lifelong Learning Institute), in discussion with author, December 13, 2024.

15. Seth Green (dean, Graham School of Continuing Liberal and Professional Studies, University of Chicago), in discussion with author, August 24, 2024.

16. Green, discussion.

17. Jason Gonzales, "Retiring Workers Find New Life Through University of Colorado Denver Program," Chalkbeat Colorado, June 26, 2023, https://www.chalkbeat.org/colorado/2023/6/26/23771788/change-makers-program-university-of-colorado-denver-program-retirees-retiring-workers/.

18. Marc Freedman (founder, CoGenerate), in discussion with author, March 11, 2025.

19. Freedman, discussion.

20. Jane Lodato, in discussion with author, April 24, 2025.

21. Celine Abecassis-Moedas (codeveloper, Longevity Leadership Program), in discussion with author, September 24, 2024.

22. Abecassis-Moedas, discussion.

23. Avivah Wittenberg-Cox (codeveloper, Longevity Leadership Program), in discussion with author, June 24, 2024.

Chapter 4: Workplaces Reimagined
for Longer Lifespans

1. "Older Workers Will Fill 150 Million More Jobs Globally by 2030, Exceeding a Quarter of the Workforce in High-Income Countries," Bain & Company press release, July 13, 2023, https://www.bain.com/about/media-center/press-releases /2023/older-workers-will-fill-150-million-more-jobs-globally-by-2030 -exceeding-a-quarter-of-the-workforce-in-high-income-countries/.
2. Michael Clinton, "The Seismic Shift That's About to Change the American Workplace," *Esquire*, February 13, 2024, https://www.esquire.com/news-poli tics /a46754477/american-workplace-change-older-employees/.
3. Michael Clinton, "Seismic Shift."
4. Anu Madgavkar, Marc Canal Noguer, Chris Bradley, Olivia White, Sven Smit, and T.J. Radigan, *Dependency and Depopulation? Confronting the Consequences of a New Demographic Reality* (McKinsey Global Institute, January 2025), https://www.mckinsey.com/mgi/our-research/dependency-and-depop ulation-confronting-the-consequences-of-a-new-demographic-reality.
5. Mike Mansfield (CEO, ProAge.org), in discussion with author, October 4, 2024.
6. Mansfield, discussion.
7. Mansfield, discussion.
8. Mitchell Stevens (professor, Stanford), in discussion with author, March 20, 2025.
9. Stevens, discussion.
10. Kerry Hannon (author), in discussion with author, April 25, 2025.
11. Hannon, discussion.
12. Patrick Lynch, "How Michelin Developed an Innovative Talent Development Program Using Career Managers," LinkedIn, December 21, 2015, https://www .linkedin.com/pulse/how-michelin-developed-innovative-talent-development -program-lynch/.
13. Hannon, discussion.
14. Lyndsey Simpson (founder, 55/Redefined Group), in discussion with author, April 16, 2025.
15. Simpson, discussion.

16. Richard Fry and Dana Braga, *The Growth of the Older Workforce*, Pew Research Center, December 14, 2023, https://www.pewresearch.org/social-trends/2023/12/14/the-growth-of-the-older-workforce/.

17. *The Midcareer Opportunity: Meeting the Challenges of an Ageing Workforce*, OECD and Generation: You Employed, Inc., October 9, 2023, https://doi.org/10.1787/ed91b0c7-en.

18. Lyndsey Simpson (founder, 55/Redefined Group), in discussion with author, November 29, 2025.

19. "Aging," U.S. Department of Health and Human Services, last modified April 27, 2022, https://www.hhs.gov/aging/index.html.

20. "Re-Imagineers: Jeanne Noonan's Personal Reinvention from Media Maven to Design Dynamo," ROAR forward, June 19, 2024, https://roarforward.com/re-imagineers-jeanne-noonan/.

21. "Re-Imagineers: Jeanne Noonan's."

22. Simon Chan (longevity strategist), in discussion with author, February 20, 2025.

23. Chan, discussion.

24. Kevin Delaney (CEO, Charter), in discussion with author, January 10, 2025.

25. Delaney, discussion.

26. "State Pension Age Timetable," Department for Work & Pensions, last modified May 15, 2014, https://www.gov.uk/government/publications/state-pension-age-timetable/state-pension-age-timetable.

27. Centre for Sustainability and Structural Policy and the Division for Economic Policy, *Pension Projection Exercise 2021 Country Fiche Denmark*, Ministry of Finance, September 2020, https://economy-finance.ec.europa.eu/system/files/2021-05/dk_-_ar_2021_final_pension_fiche.pdf.

28. Anuradha Mukherjee, "Denmark's Retirement Age Is Going Up to 70 by 2040—Will Others Follow?" *The HR Digest*, May 26, 2025, https://www.thehrdigest.com/denmarks-retirement-age-is-going-up-to-70-by-2040-will-others-follow/.

29. Par Maetva, "Signing of the 50+ Employment Charter," Groupe Adéquat, May 31, 2024, https://www.groupeadequat.com/signature-de-la-charte-emploi-50/?lang=en.

30. Avivah Wittenberg-Cox, "CEOs Get Serious about Longevity Leadership—in France," *Forbes*, February 1, 2024, https://www.forbes.com/sites/avivahwittenbergcox/2024/02/01/ceos-get-serious-about-longevity-leadership--in-france/.

31. "For All Generations Program," L'Oréal Groupe, accessed May 13, 2025, https://www.loreal.com/en/commitments-and-responsibilities/for-the-people /seniors/.

32. Clinton, "Seismic Shift."

33. Bruce Horovitz, "Companies Embrace Older Workers as Younger Employees Quit or Become Less Reliable," *Time*, December 20, 2021, https://time.com /6129715/age-inclusive-workplaces/.

34. Bradley Schurman and Tamsen Fadal, "How Companies Can Support Employees Experiencing Menopause," *Harvard Business Review*, January 11, 2024, https://hbr.org/2024/01/how-companies-can-support-employees-expe riencing-menopause.

35. Yvonne Sonsino (former lead, Mercer), in discussion with author, March 13, 2025.

36. Sonsino, discussion.

37. Avivah Wittenberg-Cox, "Flexibility for All: Unilever's Vision of the Future of Work," *Forbes*, May 24, 2021, https://www.forbes.com/sites/avivahwittenberg cox/2021/05/23/flexibility-for-all--unilevers-vision-of-the-future-of-work/.

38. Yvonne Sonsino, *Living Longer, Better: Understanding Longevity Literacy* (World Economic Forum and Mercer), June 2023, https://www.mercer.com /assets/be/en_be/shared-assets/global/attachments/pdf-2023-wef-living-longer -better-understanding-longevity-literacy.pdf.

39. TPC Team, "What Type of Portfolio Career Is Right for You?" the Portfolio Collective, accessed November 7, 2025, https://portfolio-collective.com /content/articles/what-type-of-portfolio-career-is-right-for-you/.

40. Ben Legg (founder, portfolio-collective.com), in discussion with author, April 25, 2025.

41. Legg, discussion.

42. "Two-Thirds of Workers Taking on Multiple Jobs, Study Finds," *People Management*, December 17, 2021, https://www.peoplemanagement.co.uk /article/1743090/two-thirds-workers-taking-multiple-jobs-study-finds.

Chapter 5: How Do You Launch a New Career or Become an Entrepreneur at 50 or Beyond?

1. Norman Miller, email message to author, November 21, 2023.

2. Miller, email.

3. Miller, email.

4. Ezra Greenberg, Erik Schaefer, and Brooke Weddle, "Tradespeople Wanted: The Need for Critical Trade Skills in the US," McKinsey & Company, April 9, 2024, https://www.mckinsey.com/capabilities/people-and -organizational-performance/our-insights/tradespeople-wanted-the-need-for -critical-trade-skills-in-the-us.

5. Ben Cohen, "The Investor Betting on People in Their 50s and 60s—Because Older Is Better," *Wall Street Journal*, February 7, 2025, https://www.wsj.com /business/entrepreneurship/the-investor-betting-on-people-in-their-50s-and -60sbecause-older-is-better-f19fd19b.

6. Ron Minutella, email message to author, December 21, 2023.

7. Minutella, email.

8. Minutella, email.

9. Yolanda Taylor, email message to author, December 21, 2023.

10. Taylor, email.

11. Peg Pardini, in discussion with author, February 16, 2025.

12. Luciano Bernardini de Pace, in discussion with author, July 12, 2024.

13. Bernadini de Pace, discussion.

14. Wendy Wright, email message to author, August 19, 2024.

15. Wright, email.

16. Adam Weiss, email message to author, January 23, 2024.

17. Weiss, email.

18. Alison Matz, email message to author, October 13, 2024.

19. Matz, email.

20. Barbara Kotlikoff, email message to author, October 13, 2024.

21. Kotlikoff, email.

22. Kerby Meyers, "Entrepreneurs of a Certain Age, in This Uncertain Time," Kauffman Foundation, August 5, 2020, https://www.kauffman.org/currents /entrepreneurs-of-a-certain-age-uncertain-time/.

23. Thomas Schøtt, Edward Rogoff, Mike Herrington, and Penny Kew, *Special Topic Report 2016–2017: Senior Entrepreneurship*, Global Entrepreneurship Monitor, 2017, https://gemconsortium.org/report/gem-2016 -2017-report-on-senior-entrepreneurship.

24. Jeanne Hedden Gallagher, "Older Entrepreneurs as Successful as Their Younger Counterparts, Study Reveals," Rensselaer Polytechnic Institute, April 6, 2020, https://news.rpi.edu/content/2020/04/06/older-entrepreneurs -successful-their-younger-counterparts-study-reveals.

25. Elizabeth Isele and Edward G. Rogoff, "Senior Entrepreneurship: The New Normal," *Public Policy & Aging Report* 24, no. 4 (2014): 141–147, https://doi.org/10.1093/ppar/pru043.

26. Kumar Mehta, "Older Entrepreneurs Outperform Younger Founders—Shattering Ageism," *Forbes*, August 23, 2022, https://www.forbes.com/sites/kmehta/2022/08/23/older-entrepreneurs-outperform-younger-foundersshattering-ageism/.

Chapter 6: Got Money?
Can We Fund a 100-Year Life?

1. "Life Expectancy for Social Security," Social Security Administration, accessed April 24, 2025, https://www.ssa.gov/history/lifeexpect.html.

2. "Get the Facts on Older Americans," National Council on Aging, June 1, 2024, https://www.ncoa.org/article/get-the-facts-on-older-americans/.

3. "Survey of the Retirement Landscape: Participant Perspectives," Voya Investment Management, June 1, 2025, https://individuals.voya.com/insights/education/survey-retirement-landscape-participant-perspectives.

4. "Survey of the Retirement Landscape."

5. Cyrus Bamji (chief strategy and communications officer, Alliance for Lifetime Income), in discussion with author, March 11, 2025.

6. Katy Knox (president, Bank of America Private Bank), in discussion with author, June 16, 2025.

7. Knox, discussion.

8. Knox, discussion.

9. Russell T. Hill, *Optimizing Longevity: A Road Atlas for a Happier, Less Predictable Life* (Longevity Action Publishing, 2024), 217.

10. Robert Shapiro and Luke Stuttgen, *The Peak Boomers Impact Study: Executive Summary*, Retirement Income Institute and Alliance for Lifetime Income, April 2024, https://www.protectedincome.org/wp-content/uploads/2024/04/Peak-Boomers-Econ-Impact-Study-EXEC-SUMM-ALI-RII-Shapiro-Stuttgen-EMBARGOED-Apr-18-2024-041624.pdf.

11. Jason J. Fichtner, "The Peak 65 Zone is Here—Creating a New Framework for America's Retirement Security," Retirement Income Institute and Alliance for Lifetime Income (January 2024): 1, https://www.protectedincome.org/wp-content/uploads/2024/01/Whitepaper_Fichtner.pdf.

12. Robert Shapiro and Luke Stuttgen, "The Peak Boomers Impact Study: A Majority of Peak Boomers Are Not Financially Prepared for Retirement and Their Retirements Will Have Large Effects on the U.S. Economy," Retirement Income Institute and Alliance for Lifetime Income (April 2024), 2. https://www.protectedincome.org/wp-content/uploads/2024/04/Peak-Boomers-Econ-Impact-Study-EXEC-SUMM-ALI-RII-Shapiro-Stuttgen-EMBARGOED-Apr-18-2024-041624.pdf.

13. *ALI Cannex Protected Retirement Income and Planning (PRIP) Study 2024 Report*, "Chapter 1, Retirement Defined and Peak 65," Alliance for Lifetime Income, 2024, https://www.protectedincome.org/wp-content/uploads/2022/08/2024-PRIP-Chapter-1-Release-May-17-2024.pdf.

14. Bamji, discussion.

15. Bamji, discussion.

16. "Cerulli Anticipates $84 Trillion in Wealth Transfers Through 2045," Cerulli Associates press release, January 20, 2022, https://www.cerulli.com/press-releases/cerulli-anticipates-84-trillion-in-wealth-transfers-through-2045.

17. Maeen Shaban, *Family Wealth Transfer 2024*, Altrata, June 11, 2024, https://altrata.com/reports/family-wealth-transfer-2024.

18. Knox, in discussion.

19. "Policy Basics: Where Do Our Federal Tax Dollars Go?" Center on Budget and Policy Priorities, January 28, 2025, https://www.cbpp.org/research/federal-budget/where-do-our-federal-tax-dollars-go.

20. Jason Fichtner (former deputy commissioner of Social Security), in discussion with author, February 6, 2025.

21. Fichtner, discussion.

22. Fichtner, discussion.

23. *ALI Cannex Protected Retirement Income and Planning (PRIP) Study 2024 Report*, "Chapter 4, Accumulation to Decumulation," Alliance for Lifetime Income, 2024, https://www.protectedincome.org/wp-content/uploads/2022/08/2024-PRIP-Chapter-4.pdf.

24. "The Social Security Strategy: Empowering Workers and Employers in the New Retirement Landscape," *ROAR Report*, December 2024.

25. Fichtner, discussion.

26. "Prudential Launches SimplyIncome for Workplace Retirement Plans on Fidelity Investments™ Platform," Prudential news release, January 25, 2024, https://news.prudential.com/us-en/latest-news/prudential-news/2024/q1/prudential-launches-simplyincome-for-workplace-retirement-plans-on-fidelity-investments-platform.

27. Hill, *Optimizing Longevity*, 230.
28. "Secure 2.0 Act of 2022 Summary and Guidance," ADP, accessed October 1, 2025, https://www.adp.com/what-we-offer/benefits/retirement/secure-2.aspx.
29. Larry Fink, "Larry Fink's 2024 Annual Chairman's Letter to Investors," BlackRock, accessed October 1, 2025, https://www.blackrock.com/corporate /investor-relations/2024-larry-fink-annual-chairmans-letter.
30. Trenton Reed, "What Is a State-Mandated Retirement Plan?" Human Interest, last modified December 19, 2025, https://humaninterest.com/learn/articles /what-is-a-state-sponsored-retirement-plan/.
31. Gopi Shah Goda (director, Retirement Security Project), in discussion with author, September 23, 2024.
32. Goda, discussion.
33. Goda, discussion.
34. "Life Expectancy of the World Population," Worldometer, accessed April 24, 2025, https://www.worldometers.info/demographics/life-expectancy/.
35. Haleh Nazeri and Rich Nuzum, *Longevity Economy Principles: The Foundation for a Financially Resilient Future*, World Economic Forum and Mercer, January 2024, https://www3.weforum.org/docs/WEF_Longevity_Economy _Principles_2024.pdf.
36. Haleh Nazeri (lead, Longevity Economy, World Economic Forum), in discussion with author, February 24, 2025.
37. Nazeri and Nuzum, *Longevity Economy Principles*, 15.
38. Nazeri, discussion.
39. Nazeri, discussion.
40. Nazeri and Nuzum, *Longevity Economy Principles*, 14, 21, 27.
41. Nazeri and Nuzum, *Longevity Economy Principles*, 5.
42. Annamaria Lusardi and Leora Klapper, "Financial Literacy Around the World: Insights from the S&P Global FinLit Survey," data release, Global Financial Literacy Excellence Center, November 18, 2015, https://gflec.org/wp -content/uploads/2015/11/ALPrez.pdf.
43. Mark T. Johnsen (founder, WealthArchitects), in discussion with author, February 14, 2025.
44. Johnsen, discussion.
45. Johnsen, discussion.
46. Craig Lyman (faculty, Columbia University), in discussion with author, April 4, 2025.
47. Lyman, discussion.
48. Lyman, discussion.

Chapter 7: Creativity: It Should Never Stop

1. Paul Theroux, email message to author, February 10, 2025.
2. Theroux, email.
3. Theroux, email.
4. Isabel Allende, "How to Live Passionately—No Matter Your Age," TED Talk, March 2014, Vancouver, BC, 8 min. 6 sec., https://www.ted.com/talks/isabel_allende_how_to_live_passionately_no_matter_your_age.
5. Gerhard Richter website, biography, https://www.gerhard-richter.com/en/biography.
6. Sam Nichols, "Dancer Eileen Kramer, 'Longest Living Woman in NSW,' Dies aged 110," ABC Australia, November, 15, 2024, https://www.abc.net.au/news/2024-11-15/nsw-dancer-dies-age-110-eileen-kramer/104608440.
7. Theroux, email.
8. Lev Grossman, "Frank McCourt, Author of *Angela's Ashes*, Dies," *Time*, July 19, 2009, https://time.com/archive/6689006/frank-mccourt-author-of-angelas-ashes-dies/.
9. Alexandra Alter, "Questions About an Unsolved Murder Linger over 'Where the Crawdads Sing,'" *New York Times*, July 19, 2022, https://www.nytimes.com/2022/07/19/books/where-the-crawdads-sing-delia-owens-murder-investigation.html.
10. Lot 139, Christie's sale, November 30, 2006, https://www.christies.com/en/lot/lot-4816730.
11. Adam Gopnik, *The Real Work: On the Mystery of Mastery* (Liveright Publishing Corporation, 2023).
12. "How Creativity Echoes in Health," SmartWellness, September 28, 2024, https://www.smartwellness.eu/blog-en/how-creativity-echoes-in-health.
13. "Theatre and Museum Trips Linked to Living Longer," University College London, December 19, 2019, https://www.ucl.ac.uk/news/2019/dec/theatre-and-museum-trips-linked-living-longer.
14. Josh, "5 Musical Instruments for Older People to Learn," LifeConnect24, February 2, 2024, https://www.lifeconnect24.co.uk/blog/5-musical-instruments-older-people-learn/.
15. "Modern Living: Ozmosis in Central Park," *Time*, October 4, 1976, https://time.com/archive/6852180/modern-living-ozmosis-in-central-park/.
16. John-Morgan Bush (dean, Juilliard Extension), in discussion with author, February 17, 2025.
17. Bush, discussion.

18. Bush, discussion.
19. Bush, discussion.
20. Christopher Leech (director, GenSpace), in discussion with author, February 20, 2025.
21. Leech, discussion.
22. Laura Collins-Hughes, "The Next Hot Playwright? They Prefer the Ones Who Cooled Off," *New York Times*, February 10, 2025, https://www.nytimes.com/2025/02/10/theater/tent-theater-company-older-playwrights.html.
23. Collins-Hughes, "The Next Hot Playwright?"
24. "About Stagebridge," Stagebridge, accessed October 1, 2025, https://www.stagebridge.org/about-1.
25. Michael Ognibene (CEO, Talent Is Timeless), in discussion with author, August 13, 2025.
26. Anna Gardner, "A New Beginning After 60: Rosemarie's Winning Moment," Henry Street Settlement, November 1, 2024, https://www.henrystreet.org/news/latest-news/a-new-beginning-after-60-rosemaries-winning-moment/.
27. Ognibene, discussion.
28. Alex Rotas, email message to author, May 15, 2024.
29. Rotas, email.
30. Rotas, email.
31. Rotas, email.
32. Alissa Randall, email message to author, September 22, 2023.
33. Randall, email.
34. Jonathan Fisher, in discussion with author, November 19, 2024.
35. Fisher, discussion.
36. Fisher, discussion.
37. Fisher, discussion.
38. John Kneapler, in discussion with author, February 28, 2025.
39. Kneapler, discussion.
40. Kneapler, discussion.
41. Kneapler, discussion.
42. Tina Woods, "At 60 I've Become DJ Tina Technotic (and Get a Free Bus Home)," *The Sunday Times*, July 14, 2024, https://www.thetimes.com/article/i-became-a-club-dj-at-60-my-sons-think-its-great-i-rave-hn0gw75mh.
43. Don Loftus, in discussion with author, February 21, 2023.
44. Loftus, discussion.

Chapter 8: Advertising and Media in the Age of the New Longevity

1. Erica Kwok (senior VP and general manager, Estée Lauder), in discussion with author, May 21, 2025.
2. John Dick (founder and CEO, CivicScience), in discussion with author, October 17, 2024.
3. ROAR forward and National Research Group, "Meet the Re-Imagineers," paper presented to ROAR clients, Fall 2023.
4. AARP Global Thought Leadership, "The Longevity Economy® Outlook," January 30, 2020, https://www.aarp.org/pri/topics/work-finances-retirement/economics-aging/longevity-economy-outlook/.
5. David Sable (vice-chairman, Stagwell), in discussion with author, January 29, 2025.
6. Ruth La Ferla, in discussion with author, December 20, 2023.
7. La Ferla, discussion.
8. Susan Lee Colby (founder and chief creative officer, Grace Creative), in discussion with author, December 18, 2024.
9. Colby, discussion.
10. Colby, email message to author, December 19, 2024.
11. Colby, discussion.
12. Diane Epstein (executive VP, Dentsu Creative), in discussion with author, November 21, 2024.
13. Epstein, discussion.
14. Paul Woolmington (CEO, Canvas Worldwide), in discussion with author, December 2, 2024.
15. Woolmington, discussion.
16. Woolmington, discussion.
17. Charlene Weisler, "A+E Research: Why Older Adults Matter to Advertisers," MediaVillage, February 8, 2022, https://www.mediavillage.com/article/ae-research-why-older-adults-matter-to-advertisers/.
18. "New Study Shows Age Discrimination Against Older People in Global Advertising," Agediscrimination.info, August 25, 2023, https://www.agediscrimination.info/news/2023/8/25/new-study-shows-age-discrimination-against-older-people-in-global-advertising.
19. Patrick Witschi, Aparna Bharadwaj, Gaby Barrios, and Joanna Stringer, "Don't Overlook Your Mature Consumers," Boston Consulting Group, July 11, 2023, https://www.bcg.com/publications/2023/marketing-to-mature-consumers.

20. Witschi et al., "Don't Overlook Your Mature Consumers."

21. Sable, discussion.

22. Jeffrey Gottfried, *Americans' Social Media Use*, Pew Research Center, January 31, 2024, https://www.pewresearch.org/internet/2024/01/31/americans -social-media-use/.

23. Woolmington, discussion.

24. "Our Story," CADDIS Eye Appliances, accessed October 1, 2025, https:// caddislife.com/pages/about.

25. Kwok, discussion.

26. Martha McCully, "How QVC Embraced the Longevity Movement with the Age of Possibility," *ROAR Report*, June 2025.

27. "Welcome to the Silver Marketing Association," Silver Marketing Association, accessed March 7, 2025, https://silvermarketingassociation.org/.

28. Debbie Marshall (founder, Silver Marketing Association), in discussion with author, November 14, 2023.

29. Michael Clinton, "The Huge, Fast-Growing Audience That Hollywood Is Just Ignoring," *Esquire*, May 16, 2023, https://www.esquire.com/entertainment /a43895719/why-hollywood-ignores-older-audiences/.

30. Clinton, "The Huge, Fast-Growing Audience."

31. Clinton, "The Huge, Fast-Growing Audience."

Chapter 9: The Longevity Travel Era Comes of Age

1. Melissa Biggs Bradley (founder, Indagare Travel), email message to author, February 8, 2025.

2. Matt Turner, "Stats: Senior Travelers Making a Return in 2023," Travel Agent Central, March 15, 2023, https://www.travelagentcentral.com/your-business /stats-senior-travelers-making-return-2023.

3. ROAR forward and National Research Group, "Meet the Re-Imagineers," paper presented to ROAR clients, Fall 2023.

4. Beth Mcgroarty, "Industry Research: New Data on Wellness Tourism: Projected to Hit $817 Billion This Year, $1.3 Trillion in 2025," Global Wellness Institute, January 11, 2022, https://globalwellnessinstitute.org /global-wellness-institute-blog/2022/01/11/industry-research-new-data-on -wellness-tourism-projected-to-hit-817-billion-this-year-1-3-trillion-in-2025/.

5. "Defying Convention to Deepen Connections: Booking.com's Nine Predictions for Travel in 2025," Booking.com, October 16, 2024, https://news

.booking.com/defying-convention-to-deepen-connections-bookingcoms-nine-predictions-for-travel-in-2025/.

6. "Defying Convention."

7. Jen Barr, "Travel Outlook Fall 2024: Indagare's Travel Trends Survey," Indagare, accessed September 15, 2025, https://indagare.com/article/travel-trends-survey-fall-2024.

8. "Canyon Ranch Launches LONGEVITY8™: The Wellness Industry's Most Thorough and Thoughtful Program to Live Younger Longer," PR Newswire news release, August 20, 2024, https://www.prnewswire.com/news-releases/canyon-ranch-launches-longevity8-the-wellness-industrys-most-thorough-and-thoughtful-program-to-live-younger-longer-302226600.html.

9. Klara Glowczewska (executive travel editor, *Town & Country*), email message to author, February 9, 2025.

10. Biggs Bradley, email.

11. Noelle Mateer, "SBE Launches Longevity-Focused Resort Brand amid Strategic Expansion," Hotel Dive, September 17, 2024, https://www.hoteldive.com/news/sbe-launches-the-estate-longevity-hotels/727208/.

12. Jen Murphy, "Adventure Travel Is Increasingly Not Just for the Young," *Wall Street Journal*, March 26, 2024, https://www.wsj.com/lifestyle/travel/adventure-travel-older-travelers-28b4c15d.

13. *The 2025 Travel Trend Report*, Accor, March 31, 2025, https://all.accor.com/a/en/limitless/thematics/lifestyle-trends/travel-trends-2025.html.

14. Tom Hale (founder, Backroads), in discussion with author, February 4, 2025.

15. Hale, discussion.

16. James Moses (president, Road Scholar), in discussion with author, March 7, 2025.

17. Moses, discussion.

18. Moses, discussion.

19. "State of the Cruise Industry Report," Cruise Lines International Association, May 8, 2024, https://cruising.org/sites/default/files/2025-03/2024%20State%20of%20the%20Cruise%20Industry%20Report_updated%20050824_Web.pdf.

20. Fran Golden, "What's New in Cruising in 2024," *AFAR*, January 22, 2024, https://www.afar.com/magazine/top-cruise-trends.

21. Alister Punton (founder and CEO, Storylines), in discussion with author, March 17, 2025.

22. Punton, discussion.

Chapter 10: The New Longevity Medicine and Its Impact on All of Us

1. Ronjon Nag (adjunct professor, Stanford), in discussion with author, September 23, 2024.
2. Nag, discussion.
3. Eric Verdin (president and CEO, Buck Institute for Research on Aging), in discussion with author, September 12, 2024.
4. Verdin, discussion.
5. Verdin, discussion.
6. Verdin, discussion.
7. Verdin, discussion.
8. Verdin, discussion.
9. Mark Lachs (professor, Weill Cornell Medical College; director, Cornell Center for Aging Research and Clinical Care), in discussion with author, September 23, 2024.
10. Lachs, discussion.
11. Lachs, discussion.
12. "The TAME Trial: Targeting the Biology of Aging. Ushering a New Era of Interventions," American Federation for Aging Research, accessed October 1, 2025, https://www.afar.org/tame-trial.
13. Michael Leone and Nir Barzilai, "An Updated Prioritization of Geroscience-Guided FDA-Approved Drugs Repurposed to Target Aging," *Medical Research Archives* 12, no. 2 (2024): 1–12, https://doi.org/10.18103/mra.v12i2.5138.
14. Tom Rando (professor, UCLA), in discussion with author, September 13, 2024.
15. Rando, discussion.
16. Jennifer Garrison (assistant professor, Buck Institute for Research on Aging), in discussion with author, December 4, 2024.
17. Garrison, discussion.
18. Garrison, discussion.
19. Garrison, discussion.
20. "Life Expectancy of the World Population," Worldometer, accessed February 7, 2025, https://www.worldometers.info/demographics/life-expectancy/.
21. Ong Ye Kung, "A Conversation with Ong Ye Kung, Minister for Health, Singapore," interview by Esther Krofah, Asia Summit 2024, September 19,

2024, https://milkeninstitute.org/content-hub/event-panels/conversation-ong -ye-kung-minister-health-singapore.

22. Lee Li Yang, "NDR 2025: 1.3 Million Enrolled in Healthier SG, More Urged to Sign Up," *The Straits Times*, last modified August 19, 2025, https://www.straitstimes.com/singapore/politics/ndr-2025-1-3m-enrolled -in-healthier-sg-more-urged-to-sign-up.

23. *White Paper on Healthier SG*, Ministry of Health, Singapore, 2022, https://www.healthiersg.gov.sg/resources/white-paper/.

24. *Action Plan for Successful Ageing 2023*, Ministry of Health, Singapore, 2024, https://www.moh.gov.sg/others/resources-and-statistics/action-plan-for -successful-ageing.

25. Andrea Maier (professor, National University of Singapore), in discussion with author, January 14, 2025.

26. Maier, discussion.

Chapter 11: The Intersection of Medicine, Health, and Technology: It's Here.

1. Phil Newman and Christine Belleza, "Annual Longevity Investment Report 2023," Longevity Wire, accessed December 2025), https://longevity .technology/investment/report/annual-longevity-investment-report-2023/.

2. Phil Newman (founder and CEO, Longevity.Technology), in discussion with author, December 13, 2024.

3. Abby Levy (cofounder, Primetime Partners), in discussion with author, February 26, 2025.

4. Levy, discussion.

5. Newman, discussion.

6. Newman, discussion.

7. Newman, discussion.

8. Newman, discussion.

9. Peter H. Diamandis, "Billionaires Investing in Longevity," May 26, 2024, https://www.diamandis.com/blog/billionaires-investing-in-longevity.

10. Newman, discussion.

11. David Luu (founding chairperson, The Heart Fund), in discussion with author, December 3, 2024.

12. Luu, discussion.

13. Luu, discussion.

14. Luu, discussion.

15. Wendy Chapman (director, Centre for Digital Transformation of Health, University of Melbourne), in discussion with author, December 17, 2024.
16. Chapman, discussion.
17. Jennifer Schrack (director, Center on Aging and Health, Johns Hopkins University), in discussion with author, December 16, 2024.
18. Schrack, discussion.
19. Schrack, discussion.
20. Schrack, discussion.
21. René Quashie (VP, Digital Health, Consumer Technology Association), in discussion with author, January 10, 2025.
22. Quashie, discussion.
23. "The Global Wellness Economy Reaches a Record $5.6 Trillion—and It's Forecast to Hit $8.5 Trillion by 2027," Global Wellness Institute press release, November 7, 2023, https://globalwellnessinstitute.org/press-room/press-releases/globalwellnesseconomymonitor2023/.
24. Quashie, discussion.
25. Quashie, discussion.
26. Quashie, discussion.
27. Sara Czaja (director, Center on Aging and Behavioral Research), in discussion with author, January 9, 2025.
28. Czaja, discussion.
29. Czaja, discussion.
30. "Life Expectancy for Social Security," Social Security Administration, https://www.ssa.gov/history/lifeexpect.html.

Chapter 12: Improving Your Sleep to Promote Longevity

1. Erica Pandey and Carly Mallenbaum, "The Big Business of Sleep," *Axios*, January 13, 2024, https://www.axios.com/2024/01/13/sleep-tech-supplements-bedding-healthy.
2. Richard Smith, "Why We Sleep—One of Those Rare Books That Changes Your Worldview and Should Chance Society and Medicine," The BMJ Opinion, June 20, 2018, https://blogs.bmj.com/bmj/2018/06/20/richard-smith-why-we-sleep-one-of-those-rare-books-that-changes-your-worldview-and-should-change-society-and-medicine/.

3. "1 in 3 Adults Don't Get Enough Sleep," Centers for Disease Control and Prevention Archive news release, February 18, 2016, https://archive.cdc.gov /www_cdc_gov/media/releases/2016/p0215-enough-sleep.html.

4. Charles M. Morin, Bjørn Bjorvatn, Frances Chung, et al., "Insomnia, Anxiety, and Depression During the COVID-19 Pandemic: An International Collaborative Study," *Sleep Medicine* 87 (2021): 38–45, https://doi.org/10.1016/j .sleep.2021.07.035.

5. Michael H. Silber, "Who Discovered REM Sleep?" Sleep 47, no. 1 (2023), https://doi.org/10.1093/sleep/zsad232.

6. Neil Stanley, "A Short History of Sleep Hygiene," Sleepstation, last modified March 11, 2021, https://www.sleepstation.org.uk/articles/sleep-basics/sleep -hygiene/.

7. K. Spiegel, Rachel Leproult, and Eve Van Cauter, "Impact of Sleep Debt on Metabolic and Endocrine Function," *Lancet* 354, no. 9188 (1999): 1435–9, https://doi.org/10.1016/S0140-6736(99)01376-8.

8. Matt Walker, "Sleep Is Your Superpower," TED Talk, Vancouver, BC, April 2019, 19 min., 18 sec., https://www.youtube.com/watch?v=5MuIMqhT8DM.

9. Séverine Sabia, Aurore Fayosse, Julien Dumurgier, et al., "Association of Sleep Duration in Middle and Old Age with Incidence of Dementia," *Nature Communications* 12, no. 2289 (2021), https://doi.org/10.1038 /s41467-021-22354-2.

10. Alisa Bowman, "Sleep and Longevity: How Quality Sleep Impacts Your Life Span," Mayo Clinic, January 19, 2024, https://mcpress.mayoclinic.org /healthy-aging/how-quality-sleep-impacts-your-lifespan/.

11. "Size of the Sleep Economy Worldwide from 2019 to 2024," Statista, November 25, 2025, https://www.statista.com/statistics/1119471/size-of-the -sleep-economy-worldwide/.

12. Annie Atherton, "2024 Projected to Be Biggest Year Yet for Sleep Industry," Sleep Foundation, last modified January 29, 2024, https://www.sleepfounda tion.org/sleep-news/2024-projected-to-be-biggest-year-yet-for-sleep-industry.

13. Umesh Yadav, *Stress Management Market Growth Rate, Industry Insights and Forecast 2024–2031*, DataM Intelligence, last modified December 24, 2024, https://www.datamintelligence.com/research-report/stress-management -market.

14. Jenna Glover (chief clinical officer, Headspace), in discussion with author, February 12, 2025.

15. Glover, discussion.

16. Glover, discussion.

17. Djavan De Clercq, Nelly Papalambros, and Tobias Silberzahn, "Sleep on It: Addressing the Sleep-Loss Epidemic Through Technology," McKinsey & Company, June 24, 2021, https://www.mckinsey.com/industries/life-sciences /our-insights/sleep-on-it-addressing-the-sleep-loss-epidemic-through -technology.

18. De Clercq et al., "Sleep on It."

19. "DeRUCCI Wins 2024 BIG Innovation Award Best in Internet and Technology," Businesswire news release, January 10, 2024, https://www.businesswire .com/news/home/20240110488930/en/DeRUCCI-Wins-2024-BIG-Innova tion-Award-Best-in-Internet-and-Technology.

20. "ERA, the New Dawn of Sleep," Consumer Technology Association, accessed October 1, 2025, https://www.ces.tech/ces-innovation-awards/2025/era-the -new-dawn-of-sleep/.

21. Steve Sharp, in discussion with author, April 20, 2025.

22. "Stress in America™ 2020: A National Mental Health Crisis," American Psychological Association news release, October 2020, https://www.apa.org /news/press/releases/stress/2020/report-october.

23. Manjit Devgun, "5 Things You Should Know from Mind Coach Manjit Devgun," ROAR forward, February 23, 2024, https://roarforward.com/5 -things-you-should-know-from-mind-coach-manjit-devgun/.

24. Devgun, "5 Things."

25. Glover, discussion.

26. Meeta Singh (psychiatrist and sleep medicine specialist), in discussion with author, December 17, 2024.

27. Singh, discussion.

28. Singh, discussion.

29. Michael Clinton, "Why Are Americans So Bad at Getting Old?, Oprah Daily, June 21, 2023, https://www.oprahdaily.com/life/health/a44157181/why -are-americans-bad-at-getting-old/.

30. Becca Levy, *Breaking the Age Code: How Your Beliefs About Aging Determine How Long and Well You Live* (HarperCollins, 2022), 91.

31. Clinton, "Why Are Americans."

Chapter 13: Diet and Exercise: The Longevity Lifestyle

1. Peter Attia and Bill Gifford, *Outlive: The Science and Art of Longevity* (Harmony, 2023), 292.

2. Giuseppe Passarino, Francesco De Rango, and Alberto Montesanto, "Human Longevity: Genetics or Lifestyle? It Takes Two to Tango," *Immunity and Ageing* 13 (April 5, 2016): 12, https://doi.org/10.1186/s12979-016-0066-z.

3. Michael Fredericson (professor, Stanford), in discussion with author, February 22, 2025.

4. Fredericson, discussion.

5. Joan MacDonald (fitness guru), in discussion with author, May 5, 2025.

6. MacDonald, discussion.

7. MacDonald, discussion.

8. Michael Clinton, "I'm the World's Oldest Trainer. This Is How I Work Out at 82," *Men'sHealth*, October 30, 2024, https://www.menshealth.com/fitness/a62279632/tim-minnick-oldest-fitness-trainer-interview/.

9. Clinton, "World's Oldest Trainer."

10. Renee J. Rogers (scientist, University of Kansas), in discussion with author, May 6, 2025.

11. Rogers, discussion.

12. Rogers, discussion.

13. Gabrielle Lyon (author), in discussion with author, May 12, 2025.

14. Lyon, discussion.

15. Lyon, discussion.

16. Peter Attia and Bill Gifford, *Outlive: The Science and Art of Longevity* (Harmony, 2023), 292.

17. Coreyann Poly, Joseph M. Massaro, Seshadri Sudha, et al., "The Relation of Dietary Choline to Cognitive Performance and White-Matter Hyperintensity in the Framingham Offspring Cohort," *American Journal of Clinical Nutrition* 94, no. 6 (December 2011): 1584–91, https://doi.org/10.3945/ajcn.110.008938.

18. Valter Longo, *The Longevity Diet: Slow Aging, Fight Disease, Optimize Weight* (Avery, 2019), 22.

19. Valter Longo (author), in discussion with author, September 5, 2024.

20. Longo, discussion.

21. Eric Williamson (director of nutrition, Canyon Ranch), in discussion with author, February 7, 2025.

22. Williamson, discussion.

23. Williamson, discussion.

24. Williamson, discussion.

25. Attia and Gifford, *Outlive*, 321.

26. Katherine H. Saunders (obesity medicine expert), in discussion with author, April 3, 2025.

27. Saunders, discussion.

28. Saunders, discussion.

Chapter 14: Skin Longevity:
A New Frontier of Discovery

1. Martha McCully (beauty director, *Allure*), email message to author, January 31, 2025.

2. McCully, email.

3. Valerie Monroe (beauty director, *O*), in discussion with author, January 17, 2025.

4. Monroe, discussion.

5. David Kim, Ashley Wysong, Joyce M. Teng, and Zakia Rahman, "Laser-Assisted Delivery of Topical Rapamycin: mTOR Inhibition for Birt–Hogg–Dube Syndrome," *Dermatologic Surgery* 45, no. 12 (December 2019): 1713–1715, https://doi.org/10.1097/DSS.0000000000001778.

6. Anne Chang (professor, Stanford), in discussion with author, October 2, 2024.

7. Anne Lynn S. Chang, "The Genetics of Healthy Skin Aging," Stanford Medicine Alumni Day 2023, Stanford Medicine Alumni Association, May 16, 2023, 13 min., 48 sec., https://www.youtube.com/watch?v=cad_bmy-5FY.

8. Chang, discussion.

9. Zakia Rahman (professor, Stanford), in discussion with author, February 13, 2025.

10. *U.S. Cosmetics Market Size, Share & Industry Analysis, by Product (Haircare, Skincare, Makeup, and Others), by Gender (Men and Women), by Distribution Channel (Specialty Stores, Hypermarkets & Supermarkets, Online Channels, and Others), 2025–2032*, Fortune Business Insights, last modified December 22, 2025, https://www.fortunebusinessinsights.com/u-s-cosmetics-market-108012.

11. "American Society of Plastic Surgeons Reveals 2022's Most Sought-After Procedures," American Society of Plastic Surgeons news release September 26, 2023, https://www.plasticsurgery.org/news/press-releases/american-society-of-plastic-surgeons-reveals-2022s-most-sought-after-procedures.

12. Haideh Hirmand (physician), in discussion with author, May 4, 2025.

13. Hirmand, discussion.

14. Hirmand, discussion.
15. Hirmand, discussion.
16. Hirmand, discussion.
17. Hirmand, discussion.
18. Steve Dayan (author, surgeon), in discussion with author, February 24, 2025.
19. Dayan, in discussion.
20. Dayan, in discussion.
21. Dayan, in discussion.
22. Jennifer Palmer (senior vice president, Estée Lauder), in discussion with author, May 14, 2025.
23. "Secrets to Skin Longevity: Sirtuins & Skincare," interview with Nadine Pernodet by Estée Lauder blog, accessed November 15, 2025, https://www.esteelauder.com/blog-article-skin-longevity-research-dr-nadine-pernodet-interview.
24. Palmer, in discussion.
25. Palmer, in discussion.
26. Vania Lacascade (chief innovation officer, L'Oréal Groupe), in discussion with author, April 18, 2025.
27. Lacascade, discussion.
28. Lacascade, discussion.
29. Lacascade, discussion.

Chapter 15: Relationships and Community Redefined for the Longevity Era

1. Simon van Teutem, "The Global Number of People Aged 65 Years and Older Is Set to Double Within the Next Thirty Years," Our World in Data, November 14, 2024, https://ourworldindata.org/data-insights/by-2060-the-number-of-people-aged-65-and-older-will-be-more-than-four-times-what-it-was-in-2000.
2. Office of the U.S. Surgeon General, *Our Epidemic of Loneliness and Isolation*, U.S. Department of Health and Human Services, 2023, https://www.hhs.gov/sites/default/files/surgeon-general-social-connection-advisory.pdf.
3. Fan Wang, Yu Gao, Zhen Han, et al., "A Systematic Review and Meta-Analysis of 90 Cohort Studies of Social Isolation, Loneliness and Mortality," *Nature Human Behaviour* 7 (2023): 1307–1319, https://doi.org/10.1038/s41562-023-01617-6.
4. Emily Harris, "Meta-Analysis: Social Isolation, Loneliness Tied to Higher Mortality," *Journal of the American Medical Association* 330, no. 3 (2023): 211, https://doi.org/10.1001/jama.2023.11958.

5. Liz Mineo, "Work Out Daily? OK, but How Socially Fit Are You?," *Harvard Gazette*, February 10, 2023, https://news.harvard.edu/gazette/story/2023/02/work-out-daily-ok-but-how-socially-fit-are-you/.

6. Mineo, "Work Out Daily?"

7. Usama Khan, "Percentage of Singles by Age: Key Statistics," *Retirement Living*, November 14, 2025, https://www.retirementliving.com/best-senior-dating-sites/percentage-of-singles-by-age.

8. Michael Roman (community partnerships manager, Empower 60), in discussion with author, April 4, 2025.

9. Roman, discussion.

10. Alisa Bedrov and Shelly L. Gable, "Thriving Together: The Benefits of Women's Social Ties for Physical, Psychological and Relationship Health," *Philosophical Transactions of the Royal Society of London, Series B, Biological Sciences* 378, no. 1868 (2023): 20210441, https://doi.org/10.1098/rstb.2021.0441.

11. Daniel Cox, "Male Friendships Are Not Doing the Job," Institute for Family Studies, March 28, 2023, https://ifstudies.org/blog/male-friendships-are-not-doing-the-job.

12. *10 Minutes to Togetherness*, The Li.st, Berlin Cameron, and BSG, 2024, https://www.10minutestotogetherness.com/.

13. Owen Marcus, "Five Lessons from Working with Men: Transforming Men's Approach to Emotional Wellness," ROAR forward, February 14, 2025, https://roarforward.com/five-lessons-from-working-with-men-transforming-mens-approach-to-emotional-wellness/.

14. Michael Clinton, "How to Fix America's Midlife Male Friendship Crisis," *Esquire*, December 5, 2024, https://www.esquire.com/lifestyle/a63085463/americas-midlife-male-friendship-crisis/.

15. Joe Clinton, in discussion with author, March 30, 2016.

16. Marc Freedman (co-CEO, CoGenerate), in discussion with author, March 11, 2025.

17. Freedman, discussion.

18. Sarah McKinney Gibson, *Can Intergenerational Connection Heal Us?*, CoGenerate, accessed May 13, 2025, https://cogenerate.org/loneliness/.

19. "NYC Aging Gathers Over One Thousand New Yorkers to Groove in Foley Square Park," NYC Department for the Aging press release, accessed May 13, 2025, https://www.nyc.gov/site/dfta/news-reports/press-releases/pr-aging-gathers-over-1000-new-yorkers-to-groove-in-foley-square-park.page.

20. Pat Torres (elder, Indigenous community near Broome, Australia), in discussion with author, April 23, 2024.
21. Torres, discussion.
22. "Building Better Lives—Cycling Without Age," Cycling Without Age, accessed January 2025, https://cyclingwithoutage.org/.
23. Cathaleen Chen, "Why Helsinki's Young Adults Are Moving in with Seniors," *Christian Science Monitor*, January 21, 2016, https://www .csmonitor.com/World/Global-News/2016/0121/Why-Helsinki-s-young -adults-are-moving-in-with-seniors.
24. Michiel de Gooijer, "Dutch Supermarket Introduces a Unique 'Chat Checkout' to Help Fight Loneliness," Megaphone, December 19, 2024, https:// megaphone.upworthy.com/p/dutch-supermarket-introduces-a-unique-chat -checkout-to-help-fight-loneliness-rp2.
25. "39 Caregiver Statistics, Facts and Trends," HumanCare, February 27, 2025, https://www.humancareny.com/blog/39-caregiver-statistics-facts-trends.
26. Weston Ballard (founder, Goldie), in discussion with author, March 21, 2025.
27. Ballard, discussion.
28. Assaf Gad (vice president, ElliQ), in discussion with author, February 24, 2025.
29. Gad, discussion
30. Gad, discussion

Chapter 16: Here Comes the Longevity Neighborhood, Community, City, Country

1. "The US Population Is Aging," Urban Institute, accessed January 15, 2025, https://www.urban.org/policy-centers/cross-center-initiatives/program -retirement-policy/projects/data-warehouse/what-future-holds/us-population -aging.
2. *Population in Brief 2024* (National Population and Talent Division, Singapore Department of Statistics, September 2024): 4, 11, https://www.population .gov.sg/files/media-centre/publications/Population_in_Brief_2024.pdf.
3. Selena Galan, "Countries with the Largest Percentage of the Total Population Over 65 Years in 2024," Statista (October 2025), https://www.statista .com/statistics/264729/countries-with-the-largest-percentage-of-total-popu lation-over-65-years/.

4. "Longevity," National Population and Talent Division, Singapore Department of Statistics, accessed January 15, 2025, https://www.population.gov.sg /our-population/population-trends/longevity/.

5. "Public Housing," Ministry of National Development Singapore, last updated December 6, 2025, https://www.mnd.gov.sg/our-work/housing-a-nation /public-housing.

6. "Thriving Together for a Healthier Future," Health District Queenstown, accessed October 1, 2025, https://healthdistrictqueenstown.sg/.

7. Paul Ong (deputy CEO and chief strategy officer, ComSA), in discussion with author, September 16, 2024.

8. Ong, discussion.

9. "Introduction of Outpatient Flexi-Medisave for the Elderly from 1 April 2015," Singapore Ministry of Health, January 11, 2015, https://www.moh .gov.sg/newsroom/introduction-of-outpatient-flexi-medisave-for-the-elderly -from-1-april-2015.

10. "Longevi-City: Transforming Urban Living with Longevity and Wellness in the UAE," ABNewswire press release, April 4, 2024, https://www .abnewswire.com/pressreleases/longevicity-transforming-urban-living-with -longevity-and-wellness-in-the-uae_693735.html.

11. "Longevi-City."

12. *World Population Ageing 2019: Highlights*, UN Department of Economic and Social Affairs, 2019, https://www.un.org/en/development/desa/population /publications/pdf/ageing/WorldPopulationAgeing2019-Highlights.pdf.

13. Maths Lundin, *Report: Society 5.0 Strategy in Japan*, EU-Japan Centre for Industrial Cooperation, April 2018, https://www.eu-japan.eu/publications /report-society-50-strategy-japan.

14. "Fujisawa Sustainable Smart Town," The Atlas of Urban Tech, accessed October 1, 2025, https://atlasofurbantech.org/cases/jpn-fujisawa-smart-town/.

15. Juergen Voegele, "Rethinking Silver: Lessons from Japan's Age-Ready Cities," Voices, World Bank Blogs, July 15, 2022, https://blogs.worldbank.org/en /voices/rethinking-silver-lessons-japans-age-ready-cities.

16. Emi Kiyota (founder, Ibasho), in discussion with author, October 10, 2024.

17. Kiyota, discussion.

18. Kiyota, discussion.

19. "Health Innovation Neighbourhood," Newcastle University, accessed October 1, 2025, https://www.ncl.ac.uk/business-and-partnerships/investment-pro spectus/ageing-and-longevity/health-innovation-neighbourhood/.

20. Dmitry Kaminskiy, "Investing in Health: The Rise of Longevity Havens for Affluent Investors," Henley & Partners, 2023, https://www.henleyglobal.com/publications/wealthiest-cities/global-insights/investing-health-rise-longevity-havens-affluent-investors.

21. Alana Officer (unit head, Demographic Change and Healthy Ageing, WHO), in discussion with author, August 2, 2024.

22. Officer, discussion.

23. Officer, discussion.

24. John Beard (director, International Longevity Center, Columbia University), in discussion with author, August 27, 2024.

25. *Age-Inclusive American Cities*, US Conference of Mayors (USCM) Age-Inclusive Work Group, 2024, https://www.nyc.gov/assets/cabinetforolder newyorkers/downloads/pdf/Age-Inclusive-American-Cities-Guidebook.pdf.

26. Maitreyi Bordia Das, Yuko Arai, Terri B. Chapman, and Vibhu Jain. *Silver Hues: Building Age-Ready Cities*, World Bank, 2022, https://hdl.handle.net/10986/37259.

27. Cynthia Chen, Dana P. Goldman, Julie Zissimopoulos, and John W. Rowe, "Multidimensional Comparison of Countries' Adaptation to Societal Aging," PNAS 115, no. 37 (2018): 9169–9174, https://doi.org/10.1073/pnas.1806260115.

28. *Age-Inclusive American Cities.*

29. Ghazal Ahmed, "20 Cities with Highest Elderly Population," Yahoo!Finance, July 3, 2023, https://finance.yahoo.com/news/20-cities-highest-elderly-population-121605547.html.

30. Ryan Frederick (author), in discussion with author, September 24, 2024.

31. Frederick, discussion.

32. Frederick, discussion.

33. Lindsey Beagley (senior director, Lifelong University Engagement, University of Arizona, Mirabella), in discussion with author, April 17, 2025.

34. Beagley, discussion.

35. Cade Metz, "Invasion of the Home Humanoid Robots," *New York Times*, April 4, 2025, https://www.nytimes.com/2025/04/04/technology/humanoid-robots-1x.html.

36. *Innovations in Aging*, New York State Office for the Aging, 2024, https://aging.ny.gov/innovations-aging.

37. Mark Healy, "Making New York the Most Age Inclusive City in America," *ROAR Report*, March 27, 2025.

38. Healy, "Making New York."

39. Healy, "Making New York."

40. "City of Yes for Housing Opportunity," New York City Department of Planning, accessed April 14, 2025, https://www.nyc.gov/content/planning/pages/our-work/plans/citywide/city-of-yes-housing-opportunity#overview.

Conclusion

1. Ashton Applewhite, *This Chair Rocks: A Manifesto Against Ageism* (Networked Books, 2016).

2. Louise Aronson, *Elderhood: Redefining Aging, Transforming Medicine, Reimagining Life* (Bloomsbury Adult, 2021).

3. Peter Kaldes (president and CEO, Next50), in discussion with author, April 25, 2025.

4. Kaldes, discussion.

5. "Get the Facts on Older Americans," National Council on Aging, June 1, 2024, https://www.ncoa.org/article/get-the-facts-on-older-americans/.

6. Kaldes, discussion.

7. Kaldes, discussion.